The Panic Workbook

Dr Carina Eriksen is a Chartered and UK Health and Care Professions Council Registered Counselling Psychologist with an extensive London-based private practice for young people, adults, couples and families. She is also a consultant with Dynamic Change Consultants, <www.dccclinical.com>, a psychology consultancy in London, and an accredited member of the British Association for Behavioural and Cognitive Psychotherapies, having specialized at the Institute of Psychiatry. She has managed a team of psychologists, CBT therapists and psychotherapists in the NHS for several years, and she used to be an external supervisor for The Priory. She has extensive experience consulting in clinical and organizational settings in the UK and Europe. She is a visiting lecturer at several London universities. Carina is a consultant at Colet Court, St Paul's Preparatory School for boys, and she works closely with several British and international schools in London. She is actively involved in research with a specific interest in the topics of work stress and work/life balance, anxiety disorders and living with physical illness. Carina and her colleagues are often invited to present these topics at conferences in the UK and abroad. She is the author and co-author of several books, and her work has been published in prestigious international journals.

Professor Robert Bor is a Director of Dynamic Change Consultants, and Lead Clinical Psychologist in Medical Specialties at the Royal Free Hospital, London. He is a Chartered Clinical, Counselling and Health Psychologist registered with the UK Health and Care Professions Council. He is also a Fellow of the British Psychological Society and Member of the American Psychological Association. He has more than 27 years' experience consulting in clinical and organizational settings in the UK and abroad. He is a UKCP Registered Family and Couples Therapist, having specialized in Systemic Therapy at the Tavistock Clinic, London. Rob also practises cognitive behavioural therapy and is an advocate of time-limited and solution-focused therapeutic approaches. He works with children, adolescents, adults, couples, families and teams in organizations, and is the Consulting Psychologist to the Leaders in Oncology Care and to the London Clinic, both in Harley Street. He also provides psychological consultations and executive coaching to organizations such as PWC and UBS among others, in London and abroad. He is the consulting psychologist to St Paul's School, The Royal Ballet School and JFS in London. He holds the Freedom of the City of London and is a Churchill Fellow.

Margaret Oakes is a chartered counselling psychologist registered with the UK Health and Care Professions Council. She has experience of providing psychological interventions in primary care and NHS specialist services. Margaret is a consultant with Dynamic Change Consultants. Her focus in psychological consultations is to provide tailored evidence-based interventions most likely to be effective for the individual clients she works with. She has a particular interest in anxiety disorders. Margaret is also a pilot, currently operating the Airbus A320 family of aircraft for a UK airline.

Overcoming Common Problems Series

Selected titles

A full list of titles is available from Sheldon Press, 36 Causton Street, London SW1P 4ST and on our website at www.sheldonpress.co.uk

101 Questions to Ask Your Doctor
Dr Tom Smith

Birth Over 35
Sheila Kitzinger

Coeliac Disease: What you need to know
Alex Gazzola

Coping Successfully with Chronic Illness: Your healing plan
Neville Shone

Coping Successfully with Shyness
Margaret Oakes, Professor Robert Bor and Dr Carina Eriksen

Coping with Anaemia
Dr Tom Smith

Coping with Asthma in Adults
Mark Greener

Coping with Bronchitis and Emphysema
Dr Tom Smith

Coping with Drug Problems in the Family
Lucy Jolin

Coping with Early-onset Dementia
Jill Eckersley

Coping with Eating Disorders and Body Image
Christine Craggs-Hinton

Coping with Gout
Christine Craggs-Hinton

Coping with Manipulation: When others blame you for their feelings
Dr Windy Dryden

Coping with Obsessive Compulsive Disorder
Professor Kevin Gournay, Rachel Piper and Professor Paul Rogers

Coping with Stomach Ulcers
Dr Tom Smith

Depressive Illness – the Curse of the Strong
Dr Tim Cantopher

The Diabetes Healing Diet
Mark Greener and Christine Craggs-Hinton

Dying for a Drink
Dr Tim Cantopher

Epilepsy: Complementary and alternative treatments
Dr Sallie Baxendale

Fibromyalgia: Your Treatment Guide
Christine Craggs-Hinton

The Heart Attack Survival Guide
Mark Greener

How to Beat Worry and Stress
Dr David Delvin

How to Come Out of Your Comfort Zone
Dr Windy Dryden

How to Develop Inner Strength
Dr Windy Dryden

How to Eat Well When You Have Cancer
Jane Freeman

Let's Stay Together: A guide to lasting relationships
Jane Butterworth

Living with IBS
Nuno Ferreira and David T. Gillanders

Losing a Parent
Fiona Marshall

Making Sense of Trauma: How to tell your story
Dr Nigel C. Hunt and Dr Sue McHale

Motor Neurone Disease: A family affair
Dr David Oliver

Natural Treatments for Arthritis
Christine Craggs-Hinton

Overcoming Loneliness
Alice Muir

The Pain Management Handbook: Your personal guide
Neville Shone

The Panic Workbook
Dr Carina Eriksen, Professor Robert Bor and Margaret Oakes

Reducing Your Risk of Dementia
Dr Tom Smith

Therapy for Beginners: How to get the best out of counselling
Professor Robert Bor, Sheila Gill and Anne Stokes

Transforming Eight Deadly Emotions into Healthy Ones
Dr Windy Dryden

Treating Arthritis: The drug-free way
Margaret Hills and Christine Horner

Treating Arthritis: The supplements guide
Julia Davies

When Someone You Love Has Depression: A handbook for family and friends
Barbara Baker

Overcoming Common Problems

The Panic Workbook

DR CARINA ERIKSEN,
PROFESSOR ROBERT BOR
and
MARGARET OAKES

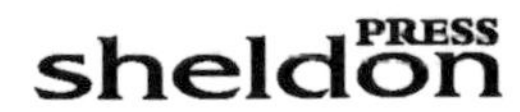

First published in Great Britain in 2012

Sheldon Press
36 Causton Street
London SW1P 4ST
www.sheldonpress.co.uk

British Library Cataloguing-in-Publication Data
A catalogue record for this book is available from the British Library

ISBN 978–1–84709–213–7
eBook ISBN 978–1–84709–214–4

Typeset by Fakenham Prepress Solutions, Fakenham, Norfolk NR21 8NN
First printed in Great Britain by Ashford Colour Press
Subsequently digitally printed

eBook by Fakenham Prepress Solutions, Fakenham, Norfolk NR21 8NN

Produced on paper from sustainable forests

This book is dedicated to the many people who have shared with us their experiences of panic attacks and anxiety. Working with them has given us insight into the ways these difficulties have an impact on thoughts, behaviour and emotions. This depth of understanding is the foundation of this self-help book, which we hope will help many others to overcome panic attacks and anxiety.

Contents

1

Why another book about panic attacks?

Anxiety is the most common psychological problem. Everyone experiences some level of anxiety in certain situations, but for some, anxiety can be a daily occurrence. It ranges from being unpleasant but temporary for some, to incapacitating and frightening for others. It can be mild or even barely noticeable but, as many people have experienced, can build up and produce panicky feelings that are intense, frightening and overwhelming. Episodes of panic can last for moments or, for some people, hours, and can occur several times a day.

Panic attacks aren't only unpleasant and debilitating, they can also be a symptom of other medical and/or psychological problems. It's therefore important to understand the mechanism by which people have panic attacks, how they can be triggered, why they sometimes persist and how best they can be overcome. Panic attacks are unwelcome enough, but for anyone who's ever experienced one, the fear of recurrence may be ever present. The reason for this is that a panic attack affects both your physiology – how your body reacts physically – as well as your thinking and feelings. The good news is that in almost all cases and situations, panic attacks can be treated and, with a clear understanding of how they happen, often prevented.

Psychological methods for treating panic attacks are well advanced, and this workbook provides a summary of the most up-to-date, tried and tested methods that many psychologists and therapists use. But other books on the subject have been published, so readers may well ask: 'Why another?' There are several reasons, and in this chapter we'll emphasize how this book differs from others.

We hope you'll find the ideas and skills we highlight useful and effective within a short time frame. Our experience with people who have difficulties with anxiety and panic attacks shows that although some books provide information about coping with specific situations, such as public speaking, going on a first date or fear of flying, they may not explain the full range of modern psychological techniques known to overcome – or at least enable you to cope with – anxiety and panic attacks.

Helping you master these techniques is the main focus of this workbook. Its purpose is to show you how to select and practise the techniques most likely to help you overcome extreme anxiety and panic attacks. We also outline the way in which panic attacks become an issue or problem in the first place, and how different people are affected by them. We describe many of the different causes or triggers of panic attacks, and readers may be surprised to learn how broad and diverse these can be.

Panic attacks and anxiety have a significant impact on the personal, family and professional lives of a substantial proportion of the adult population, as well as a proportion of children. Published research suggests that nearly 20 per cent of adults may experience high levels of anxiety in any given year, and that some of these will experience panic attacks in addition to that anxiety. This is nearly twice the number of people who experience depression, making anxiety the most commonly presented psychological problem. It may be reassuring in itself to learn this, as many people feel alone in having the unpleasant symptoms associated with extreme anxiety and panic attacks. Panic attacks can, as mentioned, affect children and young people, and can continue throughout their adult lives unless they receive specialist treatment. It's estimated that 60 per cent of people who experience attacks may also develop agoraphobia (fear of being in public places/outside), while 70 per cent of those with frequent attacks go on to develop depression.

It's fair to say that almost everyone has been anxious at some time or other, but for some there's a constant battle with anxiety in situations that give rise to unpleasant physical sensations and unwelcome and disturbing thoughts that may reinforce the feelings of anxiety. These unpleasant experiences may simply lay the foundation for further panic attacks, thereby making it a problem that appears to have no end. For some people panic attacks may be a small annoyance and something slightly inhibiting and uncomfortable; for others they may be extreme and result in avoidance of situations and ultimately referral for specialist medical and psychological treatment. This, in turn, may place strain on personal and professional lives. Clearly, then, the problems caused by anxiety and panic attacks should not be lightly dismissed.

What makes this workbook different?

This workbook takes an approach to understanding and overcoming anxiety and panic attacks that differs in five main ways from many other books on the subject:

1 It's written by a highly experienced and uniquely qualified team of psychologists who together have over 40 years' experience in treating panic attacks and helping people overcome anxiety and mood disorders, and who have published research findings in medical and psychological journals and books and spoken at conferences around the world. We're committed to helping people overcome panic attacks and to applying tried and tested methods to achieve this.
2 We're aware of and sensitive to the impact of anxiety and panic attacks in people's lives, as well as the sense of shame, embarrassment and fear they bring in their wake. Living with almost any psychological condition, such as depression, anxiety, obsessive–compulsive disorder, substance misuse or relationship problems, among many others, can affect your confidence and make you feel self-conscious. Ours aren't simply textbook ideas but are derived from the clinical experience we've already mentioned, which involves treating people with anxiety and panic attacks on a daily basis. Some of the cases we've worked with are described in this book, although naturally names and other details have been changed.
3 We approach treatment differently from some others who deal with anxiety and panic attacks, and this workbook reflects that perspective. It won't baffle you with statistics. We won't convey or focus on the idea of panic attacks as an irrational response to fear or an excessive outcome of anxiety. Nor will we dismiss

any fear you have that may seem illogical or irrational to others (and sometimes even to you!). We're more concerned with and focused on how anxiety affects you and what measures you can take to ensure you overcome it, whatever its cause. We've treated thousands of people with anxiety-related problems, and a large proportion of these have had panic attacks. We recognize how unpleasant and frightening they are for almost everyone who's experienced one, and we therefore take the problem seriously by helping you overcome it in the shortest possible time. One reason for this is that many different psychotherapeutic approaches are used in the treatment of anxiety and panic attacks. However, we're mindful of the need and importance of helping people overcome the problem as quickly as possible, starting – in face-to-face therapy – with the very first session, so that they can begin to gain confidence straightaway and, we hope, a full understanding of panic attacks and how to overcome them. This self-help book facilitates a tailored approach, built on a solid foundation of clinical practice and research. The aim is to motivate and empower you to overcome the different elements that characterize your anxiety and panic attacks.

4 We approach your anxiety and panic attacks as unique and specific issues that may differ from other people's experiences. You'll see from some of the case studies that anxiety and panic attacks affect people in many different ways. We tailor the solutions to your unique situation – we aren't exponents of a one-size-fits-all approach. When we work with people professionally, before introducing skills and ideas for overcoming panic attacks, we first listen very carefully to their experiences and stories about their difficulty. Of course, it's impossible to 'listen' to the reader of a self-help book, but we do reflect here the diverse contexts and struggles we encounter with our clients, in order to convey the complex nature of the difficulty and allow you to begin to understand and overcome your own anxiety and panic attacks.

5 The primary focus of the workbook is on the psychological skills and techniques you can apply to overcoming panic attacks. These are derived from the findings of modern psychological

research. The focus is on what you can *do* and how you can *think* about different situations to help you on your way. You'll be able to see and measure your progress at each step. Unlike some other psychological approaches, this process won't start with questions about your childhood and early upbringing, even though your earlier years and experiences may have some vague, distant or even direct reference to your panic attacks. This exploration of your past may be interesting and even beneficial, but in our experience, if this becomes the main focus of psychological treatment, you won't be introduced to the skills and techniques you need to start to overcome the unpleasant experience of panic attacks as soon as possible. Almost every psychologist or therapist will ask you something about your recent or more distant past in therapy sessions, but it's not always necessary to spend many sessions addressing your past to help you overcome panic attacks. This reflects the orientation of this book, and we focus more on what causes panic attacks (so that you can identify issues and triggers in your own life), and on treating the symptoms and effects (so that you can overcome the problem as soon as possible). If you feel that more exploration of your past is necessary, it's of course advisable to undergo psychological therapy. Modern psychological approaches focus on what's happening to you now and what you can do to bring about change, rather than on developing deep insight into your situation. You may find that some of the ideas you come across in the book can even be used and applied to help you in other areas of your life that present a challenge to you. We base our ideas not only on tried and tested clinical practice but also on such modern psychological approaches as cognitive behavioural therapy (CBT) and systemic therapy. We're interested in how people experience anxiety and panic attacks and how these, in turn, affect how they relate to those around them and how they feel inside themselves. We find that there's a circular relationship between anxiety, panic attacks, embarrassment and shame. We will say more about this later.

This is a practical self-help book designed to help you, the anxious person who has panic attacks (or a person who's affected by or related to someone with shyness or panic attacks), to gain confidence in the proven techniques and skills needed to overcome them. It will engage you in reflection and encourage you to try out new skills and tasks. It will also help you develop an understanding of your own way of thinking about anxiety and enable you to select and try out the psychological techniques likely to help you overcome panic attacks. At various points in each chapter you'll find 'Stop & think' exercises – these are designed to help you apply the information and techniques to your own situation.

As a further point of distinction from some other methods and books on anxiety and panic attacks, we've tried to avoid presenting a fixed menu of methods to overcome the problem. The main emphasis is on helping you acquire a comprehensive clinical and psychological understanding of anxiety and panic attacks and how best to resolve them. This improves the likelihood of successfully reducing panic attacks and increases your active engagement in the relevant issues. The book is structured so that you'll be empowered to confront the general, as well as the more unique and idiosyncratic, characteristics of your anxiety and panic attacks.

In clinical settings we sometimes meet people who find that taking the first step of seeking counselling for panic attacks has been too big a challenge, or who don't quickly achieve the results they wanted. If the behaviour you're trying to change has not shifted, in spite of your efforts, it's worth re-examining the nature of your difficulties once again, rather than concluding that there must be something more serious or untreatable about you – which is unlikely to be the case. We therefore encourage readers who don't feel they've made progress in the past to take a fresh look at what they're experiencing. There are numerous ways to treat panic attacks, and these aren't confined or restricted to psychological methods. Medical treatments also exist, as well as complementary techniques and methods such as homeopathy, acupuncture, meditation and aromatherapy, among others, that can be applied in addition to psychological therapy. Indeed, given the range of effective treatments now available, almost everyone should benefit and improve, and the majority of people who have panic attacks should be able to overcome them. If success has not come in the way you'd hoped, there may be several possible reasons:

- Without individual preparation and assessment, it can be difficult to identify the techniques most likely to work for your anxiety and panic attacks.
- You may be trying to use too many of the techniques you've come to understand, or not selecting those best suited to you.
- If you've attended a group for helping you overcome anxiety and panic attacks, it may be that some of the techniques most likely to work for you haven't been included.
- For some people, the amount of information they may have been given about the nature of their panic attacks may be too much, and inadvertently may have increased their fear and anxiety of their condition.
- Your difficulty with panic attacks may be being 'driven' by another issue or problem, which may need to be identified and treated in the first instance.
- It's possible that you may not be experiencing classic panic attacks. An effect of this may be that some of the skills and techniques you've learnt may not work for you yet. It's therefore important not only to keep motivated to overcome your panic attacks but to seek more specialist help from your GP and/or a psychologist or therapist, who may be able to help shed more light on your particular condition and suggest the best possible way to treat it.

Some people who experience anxiety and panic attacks prefer to work with a counsellor, therapist or psychologist to help them achieve their goals. If this is the case, this book may be a useful companion in that context. For a few readers, taking the step of contacting a trained professional is in itself stressful and anxiety provoking. You may feel inhibited through worry about how you'll come across and present yourself, and anxiety that you may be 'labelled' as having a psychological problem. If this is the case, we hope that some of the ideas covered in this book will help you either take that first step or start some of the therapeutic journey on your own. By reading this book you'll have an understanding of your own anxiety and panic attacks and how they affect you, and will be able to identify the techniques most likely to work for you. You'll then be able to concentrate on putting these into practice. It's important to undertake an individual assessment of your anxiety and panic attacks rather than assume that everyone who experiences them is alike. Should you be seeing a therapist, you can also use this book between sessions to help you practise what you've learnt.

If you're working through this book on your own or with help from a friend or relative, there are some things you can do to make the time and effort you invest as rewarding as possible. A good starting point is to decide when and where you'll work with this book. Choose a time and place when you'll be able to read and think comfortably. You may find it useful to make regular short appointments with yourself and write these in your diary or electronic calendar. Remember that learning new skills and techniques takes regular practice, so half an hour a day for a week or two might be more effective than a two-hour 'blitz' at the weekend. If you're experiencing frequent and intense panic attacks, it may be helpful to have a first read-through of the book without completing any exercises, to gain insight and understanding of the problem. You can then go back to the chapters and sections you think could be most helpful to overcome some of the unpleasant symptoms in a short time frame and to start to gain confidence and mastery of the problem. You may also find it helpful to have a notebook to hand as you work through this book. We've already mentioned the 'Stop & think' exercises, which are labelled like this:

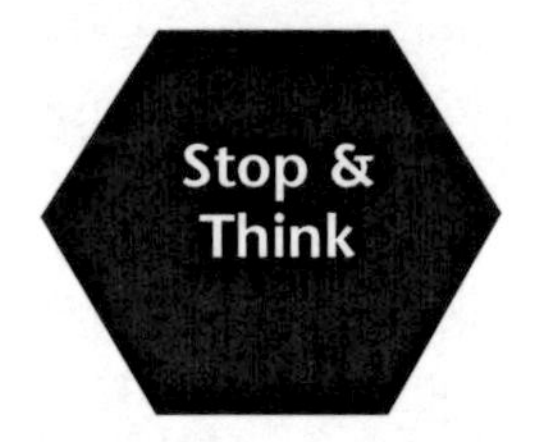

It may be tempting to skip these exercises, but we'd encourage you to spend time doing them. They're specifically designed to help you reflect on the material in this book and practise the techniques we describe. Use your notebook to record your reflections and help with practice.

In modern psychological therapy you should feel engaged in understanding and dealing with panic attacks. You're unlikely to benefit by simply reading about what may cause them: treating and overcoming them requires some work on your part, and we hope you'll find this interesting and rewarding.

As anxiety and panic attacks vary so widely, no one book can cover everything everyone needs. Once you've been introduced to the psychological techniques that we outline here, and tried them out for yourself, you may also need to use other sources of information, such as those listed in 'Other sources of help'. If you feel that progress is limited, it may be advisable to seek professional help at the earliest opportunity so that your circumstances may be more fully assessed and treated.

What's in the rest of this book

The rest of this book contains information, techniques to practise, and advice. Not all of this will be useful to everyone, but you'll find guidance on how to select and try the techniques most likely to work for you. The book is almost entirely practical in its focus, oriented to helping you first understand the source or cause of your anxiety and panic attacks from a psychological perspective. Through the case studies, it describes in detail the different presentations of anxiety and panic attacks, helping you recognize how your own difficulty with these problems affects you. It then goes on to highlight the wide variety of potential triggers that must be identified and treated to overcome panic attacks. Chapters 6, 7, 8 and 9 cover the information, skills and techniques you'll need to begin formulating your own individual treatment plan.

We've tried to write in a user-friendly and jargon-free style. A criticism levelled at psychologists is that we sometimes use terms and concepts unfamiliar to many people. We've tried to avoid 'psychobabble' and instead to focus on what's practical and usable. Although if treatment is to be effective it's helpful to understand something about the background and causes of anxiety and panic attacks, we try to avoid using terms and language that may seem alienating or unfamiliar.

Briefly, here's what each further chapter contains:

Chapter 2 describes how common panic attacks are in the general population. It also covers how panic attacks are similar to, and also different from, other anxiety disorders. There's some focus on the relationship between panic attacks and agoraphobia and depression. Crucially, we also address who's most affected and what people most fear about panic attacks. This chapter also describes both how people can be affected by panic attacks and the situations that have caused them, which will help you gain insight into your problem.

Chapter 3 looks at what causes and/or maintains panic attacks. Shame, embarrassment, fear of fear, underlying psychological issues, over-breathing (hyperventilation), fear of medical consequences or damage to your health – these and related issues may give rise to panic attacks. The focus of this chapter is on highlighting a variety of psychological causes, enabling you to begin processing and mapping out the problem in your case. This will allow for a deeper understanding of the psychological issues.

Chapter 4 provides clinical examples of cases. The aim is to provide a realistic illustration of panic attacks to reassure you that your experience may be similar to others'. It will also ask you to focus on your own panic, which may essentially be unique and slightly different from someone else's experience of it.

Chapter 5 looks at a major factor in why panic attacks may continue or recur – what psychologists call a 'failed solution'. For example, some people may avoid places or situations where a panic attack occurred in the past. Although this may provide short-term relief and feelings of being safer, it may actually intensify some of the symptoms of anxiety by prolonging and emphasizing it, as well as increase the risk of developing agoraphobia. This chapter again uses case studies to help explain this and help you understand why your attempted solution may have failed.

Chapter 6 introduces practical techniques and exercises that will help you work with what you *do* when you feel anxious, which is a fundamental part of learning to manage your anxiety and panic. For example, it covers how to start building your confidence in situations that trigger your panic. Again using case studies, it illustrates how to apply these techniques and encourages you to use them in the way most likely to manage your unique panic.

Chapter 7 describes several techniques to help you reduce physical tension and the bodily signs of anxiety. These will help you gain a sense of control over those unpleasant sensations and enable you to feel more confident emotionally. The techniques will also show you that you can cope with difficult situations. The chapter first focuses on relaxed, controlled breathing before moving on to teach you how to release physical tension and relax your body and mind. Learning how to control physical symptoms of anxiety is an effective skill that will help you stay on top of your panic.

Chapter 8 starts by listing a number of common worries likely to make us think in a way that makes our panic worse. The aim is to encourage you to start examining your own thinking so that you can begin the process of managing your fears. Another key aspect of overcoming your panic is to learn how to focus less on bodily sensations so that you can build a more balanced and perhaps more accurate picture of your physical wellbeing. Learning to focus your attention on what's happening outside of yourself, instead of what's happening inside, will help you become less focused on your body and feel more confident and secure about common bodily sensations.

Chapter 9 contains skills and techniques for working with how what you *think* may contribute to your struggle with panic and even help maintain it. Learning to identify what you think and its impact on how you feel can be fundamental to understanding and managing panic, so this chapter contains practical and straightforward techniques to challenge how you feel and to change what you do.

Chapter 10 attempts to show friends and relatives how to support someone who becomes anxious and has panic attacks, using the techniques we describe in this workbook. Many of our clients describe how difficult it can be for others to understand how to help them, but relatives and friends can become compassionate allies in helping you overcome your difficulties.

We wish you luck in overcoming anxiety and panic attacks, and hope you enjoy working through this book. You've already taken the first step towards understanding and overcoming your fear, and this motivation will add to the likelihood of success.

2
What is panic?

It's almost impossible to talk about panic without first considering the broader problem of anxiety and fear. This is because panic attacks are seen as a sub-group and phenomenon associated with anxiety and fear, even though they're not necessarily the same thing. Everyone feels anxious in certain situations or anticipation of them, but pervasive and more persistent forms of anxiety that lead to physical reactions, such as palpitations, hyperventilating, tremor, as well as thoughts turning to catastrophic outcomes, can provoke distressing feelings and lead to panic attacks. This chapter describes the relationship between fear, anxiety and panic attacks, and helps you map your individual situation as a first step towards selecting various techniques that will help you overcome your problem.

What is anxiety, and when can it become a panic attack?

Anxiety is a normal response to fear and can range from mild or almost unnoticeable feelings of nervousness to overwhelming and incapacitating terror. Everyone has some memory of what it felt like the last time they felt anxious. Almost everyone will recount one or more of the following sensations or symptoms: increased alertness or mental focus – usually on the thing or situation we feel threatened by; increased heart rate; mild sweating and what feels like raised body temperature; shallower and more rapid breathing; dry mouth and tightness in the throat; sometimes a sudden urge to visit the bathroom or the sensation that we're going to vomit; racing thoughts – usually focused on trying to get away from the situation; and 'activation' as adrenalin is released into the blood, which may make us feel 'hyper'.

Panic attacks are less common than general anxiety, but as we shall see, they reflect an intensification of anxiety and can occur for a range of reasons if anxiety is left unchecked. Panic attacks occur when we experience intense fear, sometimes quite suddenly and with little or no warning. The unpleasant and intense feelings usually last for only a short time – perhaps no more than ten minutes – but can leave you feeling drained and tired for considerably longer. They're characterized by a feeling that something truly awful is about to happen to you or is already happening. It can feel as though you may go crazy, have a heart attack or do something that will bring unwarranted attention on you and be shameful and embarrassing. Symptoms are similar to anxiety but are usually much more sudden and extreme. They include the sensation of a pounding heart; feeling out of control; rapid breathing or panting; nausea; a need to escape from the situation as a matter of urgency; the need to visit the bathroom; tingling in your fingertips; sweating; tremor or feeling shaky; a sense of foreboding and feeling strange inside yourself, as if you're not really there.

People who have panic attacks may have extreme levels of anxiety, either in particular situations or merely thinking about them, as if they were a significant yet pending danger or threat. This can be very difficult for those concerned and others because it makes everyday situations uncomfortable and may restrict and interfere with their lives. Research shows that it's often our response to feeling anxious that keeps it going or makes it even worse, and can produce panic attacks.

What triggers panic attacks?

Panic attacks can occur in specific and well-defined situations, such as before or during an examination, when flying, or seemingly out of the blue when shopping. They can also affect some people's confidence in a much broader range of contexts and cause them embarrassment and general unease. They may fear that they will have a panic attack and, as a consequence, avoid or withdraw from important work and social situations, such as business meetings, going to parties and other socializing. Avoidance or withdrawal may also occur when they need to move on in their lives, such as through attending job interviews. General unease can be among the symptoms experienced across a range of situations.

As we've said, in extreme circumstances panic attacks, or a fear of experiencing them, can lead to withdrawal from social situations. This can affect your capacity to form and maintain relationships; your ability to give – and receive – emotional and social support to or from friends and family; and can damage careers, spoil holidays and put relationships under stress.

Panic attacks are triggered by many different fears and problems: no two people are completely alike in this regard. People who experience them may have unique and specific causes of their difficulty, but they all share a problem that manifests itself in one way: they feel unable to control the symptoms of anxiety, worry and fear, which produce changes in thoughts (cognitions) as well as reactions (behaviour, mostly relating to bodily reactions). While reading through this chapter and the case studies, you'll become aware of the diverse nature of the problem and the impact that panic attacks have on people from many different backgrounds.

Many people who have panic attacks want to know how they come to experience worry and anxiety in the first instance. This is a good question, because worry and anxiety often produce panic attacks even though these are by no means the only causes. Therefore understanding anxiety is a useful way to shed light on how people come to have panic attacks. But while anxiety may be uncomfortable and unwelcome, we should not always think of it as indicating a psychological problem. Indeed, the opposite may be the case: scientists have argued that anxiety may actually be necessary in order to help protect us individually and to preserve our species. It alerts us to, and activates us in the face of, danger or threat.

Humans have the capacity to think, perceive, reflect, conceptualize and communicate. Even from a young age, we can begin to experience worries – and sometimes high levels of anxiety – about things that have happened to us. Perhaps an infant has become distressed by being separated from a parent, or a child anxious at the prospect of going to school. As we mature, we become aware of more experiences and demands in our lives and increasingly we may also become anxious about things that haven't yet happened to us. This is called 'anticipatory anxiety' and can remain with us throughout our lives. We may feel threatened and come to imagine what could go wrong (and may distort the level of challenge), or perhaps experience vulnerability and isolation in a given situation. Worry may extend to a fear of getting things wrong, not being sufficiently prepared for a situation, experiencing shame or embarrassment or even worrying about whether we'll survive a situation.

Many of these thoughts are anxieties about our ability and capacity to cope, keep calm and confident, and to succeed. They're part of the human condition, and few people are completely free of these feelings. These anxieties that we carry with us have evolved with us and are associated with survival and adaptation. As a species, we've evolved rather quickly and, in contrast to other species, our social development has done so rapidly, which often gives rise to a number of specific problems. A good example is that humans haven't naturally evolved to fly and our bodies and sometimes our thoughts can find the experience very challenging. Nonetheless, every day millions of people throughout the world take to the skies. Even though air travel is commonplace for many people, the experience or even anticipation of it can trigger significant fears and anxieties – and a proportion may have panic attacks either just thinking about flying or when on board an aircraft. Being high above the ground, flying at great speed and being in an enclosed and pressurized aircraft cabin where there may be restrictions on when we can eat or move around, can induce anxieties and panic attacks in even the most well-adjusted people. Many airline passengers' thoughts turn to fears about safety and survival. Almost everyone has a strong innate desire to survive, and anxiety may be aroused and panic attacks triggered when we feel that our survival may be threatened.

It's important to note that these fears may be regarded as 'irrational' by some people since our fears may be out of proportion to the actual threat. Yet it's difficult simply to switch off our thinking, however anxiety-laden it may be. This is our evolutionary and survival tendency being activated and perhaps, you may argue, being over-activated in certain situations. While it may be unwelcome or even excessive, these feelings don't usually indicate serious underlying psychological problems. However, gaining an understanding of what makes us feel anxious, what feels threatening and what can lead to our feeling out of control is an important first step in overcoming panic attacks.

Different people can be affected by stressful or anxiety-provoking situations in different ways. Think back to your schooldays to help illustrate this: perhaps you were in a class of students where a few excelled and didn't mind sitting examinations or being tested, while for others, exam time was distinctly uncomfortable, and they would have liked to avoid it. Another example is that many people express a fear of public speaking, and yet some have made a career out of doing just this. Every time you switch on the television or go to a play or film, you're exposed to people who presumably have had to overcome any fear associated with performing in public – or never experienced it in the first place. Not all feelings of anxiety automatically produce panic attacks. Everyone has at some point felt anxious about a situation, but has not necessarily experienced the unpleasantness of a panic attack. However, almost everyone who experiences a panic attack has also experienced some anxiety about a situation, even if it's worry or anxiety about experiencing high levels of anxiety!

At the heart of the issue, all fears and anxieties stem from a perceived threat to survival or a challenge to our confidence or self-esteem. Whatever the source or trigger, we fear something awful happening to us that could physically or emotionally – or both – endanger us. Our reactions to experiences that frighten us encompass what we do, what we think, our emotions and our physical responses.

We all have a strong instinctive mechanism that's designed to protect us from threat or danger, and this can become activated long before we confront or experience actual danger. Unfortunately, we often react with greater intensity to a threat than is warranted. This is because the automatic protection system may have been aroused before we've been able to appraise, reflect on possibilities and come up with an alternative assessment of what could occur. Physical reactions therefore typically occur before we notice what's happening to us. The approach we describe will help you slow down this process of automatic reaction and override some of the physical reactions you may have to anxiety and during a panic attack – as well as some of the thoughts you may have in the face of them.

Fear, on the other hand, is regarded as an *emotional* response to a perceived threat. Fear may lead us to escape or avoid a situation. Anxiety may arise in situations that may be seen as unavoidable and therefore from which the individual can't escape – it's therefore usually in relation to an anticipated state rather than a present danger.

Fear and anxiety can be differentiated in terms of (a) the intensity of feelings and reactions, (b) their duration and (c) the level of threat to the individual. Fear is generally considered to be a state that occurs over only a short period of time and in response to a specific challenge or threat. It often leads to the need or desire to get away from the threatening situation. By contrast, anxiety is regarded as more intense, often triggered or experienced in relation to an anticipated fear, and can last significantly longer.

Physical and behavioural effects

There are specific physical effects associated with anxiety. Many people who experience anxiety will describe feeling that their heart is racing (tachycardia, or palpitations), shortness of breath (dyspnoea), tension in the stomach or gut area, sweating, shaking/trembling and a fear of loss of bowel control or the need to vomit. These effects, as we will describe, are normal and are driven by the secretion of adrenalin and related hormones into the body that activate its alarm system. During a panic attack, all these physical effects are intense and leave the individual feeling vulnerable and out of control as he or she becomes acutely aware of the body's reactions to a stressor – breathing, heart rate and body temperature all appear to change rapidly. The common physical effects of high levels of anxiety and panic include:

- racing/pounding heart or generally increased heart rate;
- sweating;
- tremor, shaking or a sensation of reduced control over parts of the body;
- over-breathing, gasping for air or shortness of breath;
- tightness in the chest area and a feeling of restriction when

breathing, or the sensation of choking, discomfort or slight pain in the chest;
- sensation or fear of vomiting, nausea or discomfort in the stomach and the need to visit the bathroom urgently;
- light-headedness, dizziness or feeling faint;
- feeling out of sorts and not one's usual self, commonly referred to as a feeling of unreality or 'depersonalization';
- fear of losing control or going mad;
- profound sense of foreboding and a fear of dying;
- tingling sensations or numbness;
- changes in body temperature, often a feeling of being excessively hot or cold, or these sensations rapidly following one another.

When faced with such emotional and physical upheaval as that generated or triggered by a panic attack, it's understandable that most people who have them feel unable to engage in their normal everyday routines. They may also feel very tired after an anxiety attack as they have been in a state of crisis or hyperarousal and the body may be depleted afterwards. They may also withdraw from social contact, fearing that another panic attack may occur or that they'll embarrass or shame themselves if they lose self-control, hyperventilate or feel overcome with fear. Further effects include changes in sleeping patterns as they find it difficult to relax and enjoy normal sleep. Instead, anxiety levels are often so high that, together with the effect of adrenalin and other hormones circulating, it's difficult to settle and relax. They may also exhibit ritualistic behaviours such as shuffling, swinging a leg while seated or tapping in a nervous way. All of these and related behaviours reflect being unsettled physically as well as feeling emotionally out of control.

Emotional effects

The emotional effects of anxiety follow on from the physical. If you feel agitated, out of control, and your heart is racing and your breathing feels erratic and abnormal, it follows that many of the feelings you may have will reflect this. People affected by panic attacks will often feel high levels of tension, jumpiness, a sense of foreboding and intense worry about lurking dangers. You may be preoccupied with your thoughts and also hypervigilant in relation to everyday expenses and routines. For example, sitting in a classroom at school or going into a shop may feel like negative and unpleasant experiences if they become associated with unpleasant and unwelcome thoughts and physical sensations. You may have difficulty concentrating and become overly focused to the point of being obsessional about your fears. Everyday behaviours, such as conversing, may become difficult, and people often describe feeling trapped by their own negative and worry-laden thoughts. They come to dread situations that they associate with feeling anxious, and indeed being by themselves, as this can leave them feeling exposed to highly unpleasant feelings.

Cognitive effects

Thoughts reflect a sense of foreboding in the face of anxiety. We may not be able to focus or concentrate. We become less creative, more apprehensive, and worry about what may happen to us. It's often difficult to control these thoughts, which only reinforces the unpleasantness of the experience. Imagine feeling trapped with your thoughts and being unable to engage in everyday activities such as planning your diary, going to the gym or being able to shop.

Symptoms of anxiety may differ in terms of intensity. Not everyone has the same physical reactions, and not everyone who experiences anxiety also suffers from panic attacks. Nonetheless, many of the symptoms are common although their duration and intensity may vary. Panic attacks are often characterized by their sudden onset, and it's this, together with their unpredictable nature, that can make us feel out of control and lead to increased worry about their consequences. This in turn can make us feel that something bad or catastrophic might happen to us, such as losing control or consciousness, or dying. Again, the fear is enough to trigger panic attacks in some people, thereby establishing a vicious cycle or pattern that needs to be broken.

In the case studies below, you'll learn about the experiences of others who've experienced panic attacks, and what gave rise to them. They also illustrate the physical, emotional, cognitive and behavioural effects of panic attacks.

Duane suffered from situational anxiety that was triggered by a trip abroad:

> Duane, a 23-year-old man completing his university degree, first became aware of anxiety when going on holiday with friends during his gap year. He looked forward to independence from his parents and spending time with friends, but soon after booking his flight he became aware that he felt apprehensive and at times fearful of his forthcoming trip. He couldn't understand what had triggered these feelings, but he was aware that the thought of boarding an aircraft with friends and without his family made him feel frightened. As his travel date loomed closer, he became more preoccupied with his thoughts and fears and recognized that his sleep pattern was deteriorating. He'd lie awake at night worrying about the flight and that he might become anxious or even have a panic attack on board. Duane felt too self-conscious to tell any of his friends about his feelings, and he also chose not to share them with his family. On the day of departure he arrived late at the airport and found himself secretly hoping he'd miss the flight. But there was a delay, and he checked in and joined his friends in the waiting area.
>
> Once on board, Duane became more aware of his feelings and realized he was beginning to feel out of control. He told his friends he was feeling unwell and asked to be left alone, shutting his eyes and gripping the arm rests of his seat. He feared he was going to be sick, could feel his heart racing, and began to sweat profusely. Duane sat for the rest of the journey feeling anxious, panicky, fearful of what was happening to him and unable to communicate. As soon as he heard the captain's announcement to prepare for landing he started to feel better, became more engaged and alert, opened his eyes, and the feelings of nausea and high levels of agitation began to recede.
>
> Duane thought he'd had a panic attack but didn't tell anyone. He had difficulty understanding why it had happened but recognized that the unpleasant feelings were relieved once he felt that the perceived threatening situation had passed. Fearing a repeat experience on the return journey, Duane made excuses about needing to go home early and undertook a lengthy train and ferry journey to avoid flying.
>
> Duane didn't address his panicky feelings associated with flying when he got home, but when subsequently invited to stay with a friend in France, he visited his GP to ask for medication to help him cope with the journey. Fortunately his GP recognized that Duane had probably suffered a panic attack and that it would be beneficial to refer him to a therapist who could help him understand his feelings and reactions,

assess whether there were any underlying reasons or causes and provide skills to help him cope.

Duane attended four sessions of psychological counselling and managed to complete the trip to and from France successfully.

Miriam also experienced situational anxiety relating to travelling on the Underground:

Miriam was 42 years old when she suffered her first panic attack. She couldn't understand what was happening to her when, while queuing to buy an Underground ticket, she suddenly felt sick, agitated and that her breathing was out of control. She realized she needed to escape from the ticket hall as soon as possible and get into the fresh air. She sat on a bench for a while, trying to collect herself, while unpleasant thoughts raced through her mind. She worried that she was going to die and called a close friend, who accompanied her to the nearest A & E department. There she was examined, told that she was in no danger but that she'd suffered a panic attack. While Miriam was reassured by this, she didn't know what had caused the attack and was especially troubled by the fact that it had come on her unexpectedly and was a situation over which she had no control.

Miriam was referred to her GP, who assessed her the following day. The doctor diagnosed depression in Miriam, who'd recently lost a parent. Her mother had suffered a long illness and had succumbed to a rare neurological condition. Miriam had cared for her throughout, but it was not until a few months after her mother's death that Miriam became aware of her own feelings. Her GP pointed out that depression can sometimes give rise to anxiety, which in some people can lead in turn to panic attacks.

Miriam was referred on for bereavement counselling and, at the same time, for cognitive behavioural therapy to help her cope with her panic attacks. She made a full recovery in relation not only to these but to her low mood and bereavement as well.

Zack's panic attacks were triggered by medical treatment he was receiving:

Zack was diagnosed with testicular cancer at the age of 23. Treatment was swift and radical: he'd a testicle removed within 48 hours of diagnosis and the following week was started on chemotherapy. A week into this, Zack suffered a panic attack. His close family and friends all thought this was directly related to the emotional distress he'd experienced as a consequence of his cancer diagnosis.

> Zack was referred to a Macmillan nurse for counselling to help him gain insight into his medical condition and assist him in coming to terms emotionally with it. His nurse explained to him that, while emotional factors may have triggered his panic attack, it's common for people undergoing chemotherapy to experience high levels of anxiety and have panic attacks as a result of the treatment. Some forms of chemotherapy and the accompanying steroid treatment can have the effect of raising the heart rate, disturbing sleep patterns, interfering with appetite and weight, and making people feel physically agitated within themselves. Zack was reassured to learn this as he didn't understand what had left him feeling suddenly emotionally vulnerable. He also felt that the surgery and chemotherapy were in some ways not as bad as the panicky feelings he was experiencing while being treated and during recovery from surgery.

The reassurance Zack was given, combined with cognitive behavioural therapy skills to help cope with panic attacks, plus some medication, helped him overcome his panic attacks.

Lisa's anxiety and subsequent panic attacks were triggered by work stress:

> Lisa, a marketing manager, had recently returned to work following ten months' maternity leave. She began to experience intense headaches at work, which she thought were linked to parental sleep deprivation. One day, during a particularly stressful period at work, Lisa was on her way to a meeting when she started to feel increasingly dizzy. Her vision became blurred and her legs and hands began to shake. She recalls thinking: 'I'm going to pass out. There's something seriously wrong with me.' She managed to get herself to the Ladies', feeling afraid and exhausted. The following morning Lisa contacted her GP, who referred her to a therapist. The therapist explained that the combined stress of juggling work with being a mother, as well as sleep deprivation, may have caused a panic attack. It was a relief to Lisa to hear from a professional that she was 'doing too much' as she was actually fearful of not doing enough, either at work or at home! With the help of her therapist, Lisa was gradually able to reduce her responsibilities at work. At home she became more at ease with sharing parental care with her husband, which allowed her more time for physical exercise and seeing her girlfriends.

Naomi's anxiety had its origins in a fear that she'd be ill in front of others:

> Naomi, a 27-year-old television presenter, had seen several GPs and a neurologist before she was diagnosed with panic disorder. She initially thought the nausea and dizziness were due to travel sickness and vertigo. Recently, at a music festival she'd suddenly felt nauseous and her body had begun to tremble. Her mind was racing: 'I need to get out of the crowd', 'I'm going to be sick in front of my friends', 'I'm trapped; there are so many people here and I can't get out.' Naomi's heart rate increased; she felt hot and breathless. She decided to seek therapy shortly afterwards because the incident had led her to worry a great deal about having another panic attack, and she now felt anxious in situations that wouldn't have worried her prior to it. These included travelling by air or train or work meetings. In one of her therapy sessions Naomi talked about her fear of vomiting, recalling an incident when she was 18 when she'd been sick in front of an examiner. She'd felt ashamed because of it and had developed a fear of other situations where she'd need to perform in front of others.

Perhaps what we've presented in these case studies is similar to your own experience of anxiety or panic attacks. The cases differ in respect of what triggered the attacks and their effects, but they're all linked in terms of the symptoms the individuals experienced. This reflects what we've already highlighted as an important focus in this book, namely that panic attacks are caused or triggered by many different situations or problems. The next chapter describes in greater detail the experience of panic attacks as a further step towards helping you prepare to overcome them.

3

What causes or maintains panic attacks?

In this chapter we look at what causes panic, as the first step in learning to overcome it. We also introduce the psychological approach behind this book – cognitive behavioural therapy, or CBT – to help you get the best out of the techniques we'll describe later.

Why do I need to understand what causes panic – can't you just tell me how to stop it?

We'd love to be able to give you the answer to this unpleasant and uncomfortable problem in a single set of instructions. Unfortunately, people – and the way they experience panic – are so different that a one-size-fits-all approach is often ineffective. If you take the time to think about what may be causing your own unique experience of panic and use that understanding to select the techniques most likely to work for you, you're more likely to be successful in overcoming it.

The fact that your panic is a unique experience means that there isn't a single *cause* that's relevant to everyone either. As you work through this chapter, you may find that you can identify experiences or other factors that might explain why you struggle with panic now. That can be enlightening and, in some cases, help reduce the shame and embarrassment associated with panic by providing an explanation you might share with others. If you find that you don't understand *why* you panic now, that's all right. The most important thing to understand is how you *experience* panic now – when it's most likely to happen, the physical sensations, thoughts, behaviours and emotions associated with it. The 'Stop & think' exercises will help you explore your own version of panic.

If you can't identify the root causes of your panic but would like to, it may be that you can do this by working with a psychologist, counsellor or therapist later.

Experiences and other factors that may contribute to panic

While one of the themes of this book is that everybody's experience is different, there are factors that occur frequently in explaining panic.

Medical conditions

There are a number of medical conditions, for example asthma, cardiac conditions or allergies, that can produce the physical sensations of panic, such as a racing heart and difficulty breathing. Obviously all these require accurate diagnosis and, where appropriate, medical treatment. For this reason, anyone who experiences the physical sensations of panic for the first time, in new situations or with significantly different symptoms from previous occasions, should first seek medical attention. If medical causes are eliminated, that can be a finding many people have difficulty accepting. This is quite understandable but can mean they impose significant unnecessary restrictions on their lives. For example, someone who experiences a first panic attack while outside enjoying a walk may continue to avoid walking because she or he fears it might indicate that exercise could trigger a heart attack. This might limit their enjoyment significantly. Provided you check with your GP or other health professional about when to ask for medical investigations or what, if any, restrictions on lifestyle may be necessary, the techniques in this book will help you reduce that anxiety and manage your panic.

Inherited or genetic factors

Some of every individual's psychological and emotional characteristics are determined by their genetic makeup at birth. In part these inherited characteristics may mean we're predisposed to becoming anxious or developing a tendency to panic. If another family member has been diagnosed with panic or another type of anxiety, your risk of having a similar experience is increased. While we can't change this, it's possible to learn effective ways of coping with inherited characteristics.

Learned behaviour

Whatever characteristics we might have inherited, there are many aspects of how we feel, what we think and what we do that we learn from experience, whether as a child or as an adult. We might, for example, have seen someone have a panic attack or even a heart attack and been very scared by that. If we were to experience similar sensations ourselves at a later date, it would be understandable if we panicked then.

Stress

Various situations in our personal, professional and family lives may become stressful. When this happens, our capacity to deal with potentially frightening situations is reduced and we're more likely to think something is dangerous or frightening. Stress in any situation almost always results in physical symptoms of anxiety, such as racing heart, sweating or shaking, and interpreting these symptoms as something catastrophic is a common cause of panic.

Other psychological factors

Low mood (depression), anxiety and many other mental health issues can make it more difficult to cope with experiences that trigger anxiety. This is turn may make you more prone to panic. If this is a significant factor for you, you may find that you don't make the progress you'd like using the techniques in this book until you address other psychological factors. Depression, for example, often makes it more likely that you'll feel anxious, and it may be that working with that low mood is the most helpful way to start managing your anxiety and panic. If you feel you may be depressed, we strongly recommend that you talk to your GP or a mental health professional.

Medication

Some prescribed medication is associated with an increase in feelings of anxiety. Some may have uncommon side effects that reproduce the physical sensations of panic. If you think either might apply to you, talk to your GP or other health professional.

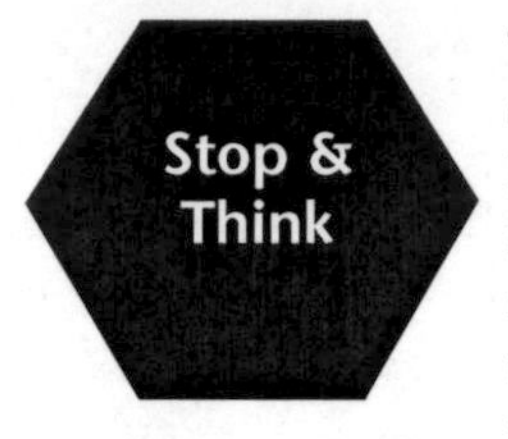

Take a few minutes to think about your own history. Do any of the factors we've listed seem to explain some of the reasons you struggle with panic? Make a note if you can identify any contributing factors – you may be able to think of things we haven't listed. This may be useful information as you work through the rest of this chapter.

You may find it useful to identify previous experiences or other factors that have contributed to your current difficulties. Many people find that they can't completely explain why they now struggle with panic. While frustrating, it isn't essential to know 'why' to get the maximum benefit from the techniques in this book. All the same, if you do want to explore the history of your difficulty, a counsellor, psychologist or therapist will be able to help.

Before we look at how to identify the important features of your individual experience of panic, we'll introduce the psychological framework behind this book: cognitive behavioural therapy. We're doing this now so you can start to look at your own difficulties in a way that will help you work with the rest of this book.

The psychology behind this book

As we have already said, the approach behind this book is cognitive behavioural therapy, or CBT. You may have seen reports on television about it as it's a very effective and popular psychological approach for many difficulties, particularly anxiety and depression. CBT is the approach recommended for use in treating panic in the UK and is effective at reducing anxiety and panic for many people.

There are three main aspects of CBT that are important to understand when working to overcome panic:

1 The link between what we think and how we feel.
2 Identifying your individual response to anxiety.
3 Modifying solutions that haven't helped.

The 'cognitive' in cognitive behavioural therapy refers to the link between what we *think* and how we feel, which often drives what we *do*. 'Behavioural' refers to what we *do* and the way in which sometimes what we do in an attempt to control or avoid panic actually keeps it going rather than being a solution. What we *do* can also influence what we *think*. That's why this approach is called cognitive behavioural therapy.

The link between what we think and how we feel

Imagine for a moment that you're at home waiting for a friend to telephone you at the end of a very stressful day. They promised to call because you've something very important to tell them and the call is the main thing you're thinking about. It gets to 11 p.m. and the phone hasn't rung. You think, 'They're not going to call because I upset them yesterday.' How would that make you feel and what would you do? You might feel very upset and have difficulty getting to sleep. You might ring another friend to complain or find that you snap at your colleagues at work the next day.

Now imagine that exactly the same thing happens: your friend doesn't call. This time, however, you think, 'I wonder if their phone has run out of charge or credit, or something happened that needed their immediate attention?' How would you feel and what would you do now? You might feel slightly concerned about them and either call them to check or decide to catch up with them tomorrow. You'd be less likely to feel upset and therefore might also spend less time thinking about the situation.

Can you see how two different ways of thinking about the same event have resulted in different feelings and actions? Unless you found out by talking to your friend or someone who knew, you wouldn't know which thought was accurate, but the way you think has had a large impact on what you feel and do. We've drawn this out in Figure 3.1 (overleaf).

This is the basis of many techniques in this book. Once you can identify what you're thinking, you can link that to how it makes you feel. Thoughts that make you feel anxious may be valid or inaccurate. If they're not absolutely valid, the most useful techniques from this book are likely to be those that show you how to challenge unhelpful thoughts and alter how you feel, improving

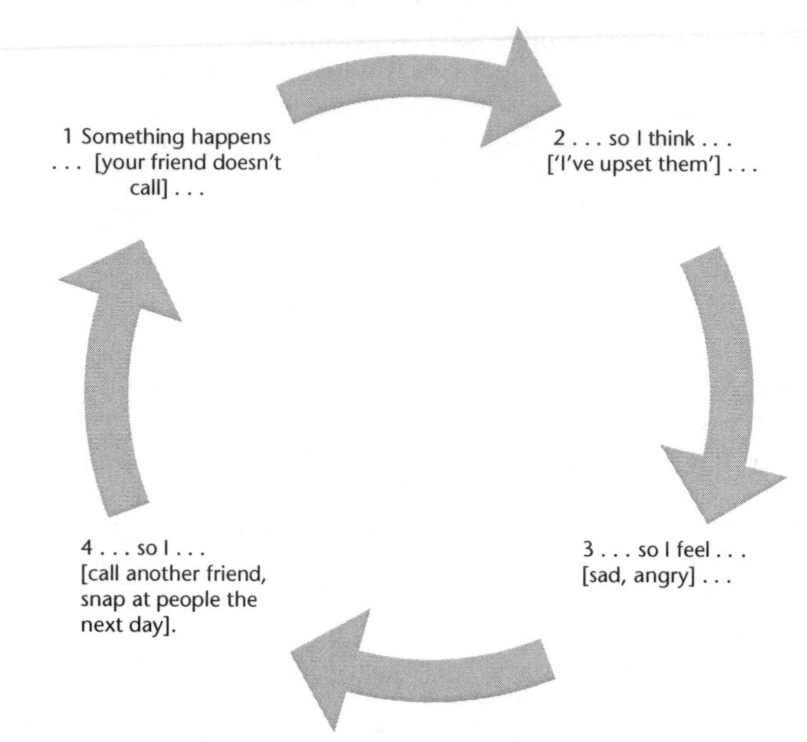

Figure 3.1 The link between what we think and what we feel and do

your confidence. If they're correct, the 'doing' techniques in the following chapters will help you change or manage the situation.

How we feel, physically and emotionally, can also have an effect on what we think, which in turn may trigger or increase anxiety. For example, if you notice that your body is tense, your heart rate has increased or your breathing has changed, you may think those symptoms indicate that something dangerous is about to happen. Once that cycle of anxiety starts, you'll almost certainly become very anxious or even panic unless you can break into it. Essentially this is a feeling that if your body feels nervous there must be something dangerous around. Working with how you think about physical sensations is often a fundamental part of managing panic.

Identifying your individual response to anxiety

Being able to describe what happens when you experience panic is important for two main reasons. First, it will help you understand more about your individual difficulties and therefore help reduce the embarrassment you may feel. Second, identifying the major themes, such as how you *think* or what you *do* when you experience panic, will help you identify which skills or knowledge in the rest of this book are most likely to help you. A useful framework for thinking about this is to notice what you feel (your emotions), what you *think*, what you *do* and how your body feels. Here's an example:

> Benito was at his father's house overseas packing some things for him. His father had been admitted to a cardiac unit with a suspected heart attack. Suddenly Benito noticed that his own heart was racing, and began to think he too might be having a heart attack. He quickly became very anxious and noticed that his heart raced even more. He also became slightly breathless and sweaty. He sat down to see if that made him feel better, and began to think about how his neighbour had described his father looking sweaty and breathless when he was taken to hospital. He became even more frightened and began to feel tingling in his limbs. Terrified, Benito rang the cardiac unit where his father was, and was rushed there by ambulance. All investigations showed no physical problem, and the medical team concluded that Benito had experienced a panic attack. Ben felt embarrassed when he left the hospital as he'd thought that his symptoms were indicative of physical illness.

This description shows all four aspects of Benito's first panic attack. Psychologists often illustrate the way we respond when shy or anxious as a 'hot cross bun', as in Figure 3.2 (overleaf).

No one can simply turn off their emotions, and it would be a very dull life if we could. When those emotions aren't helpful, however, we can work directly with what we think and do and how our body responds. Most people who struggle with panic will need to work with all three, but the skills most likely to help you are the ones that relate to the most overwhelming part of your response to anxiety.

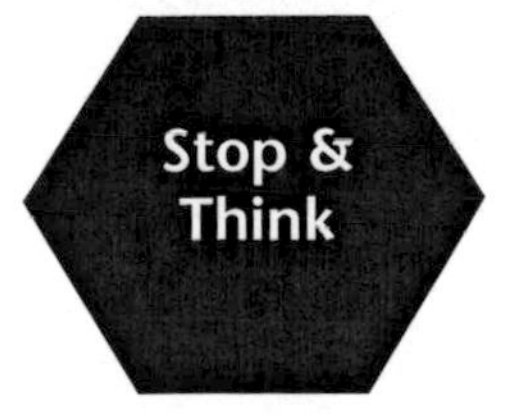

Can you draw your own hot cross bun? What do you think is the part of your response that you should work on first? Is it what you think or do or how your body reacts?

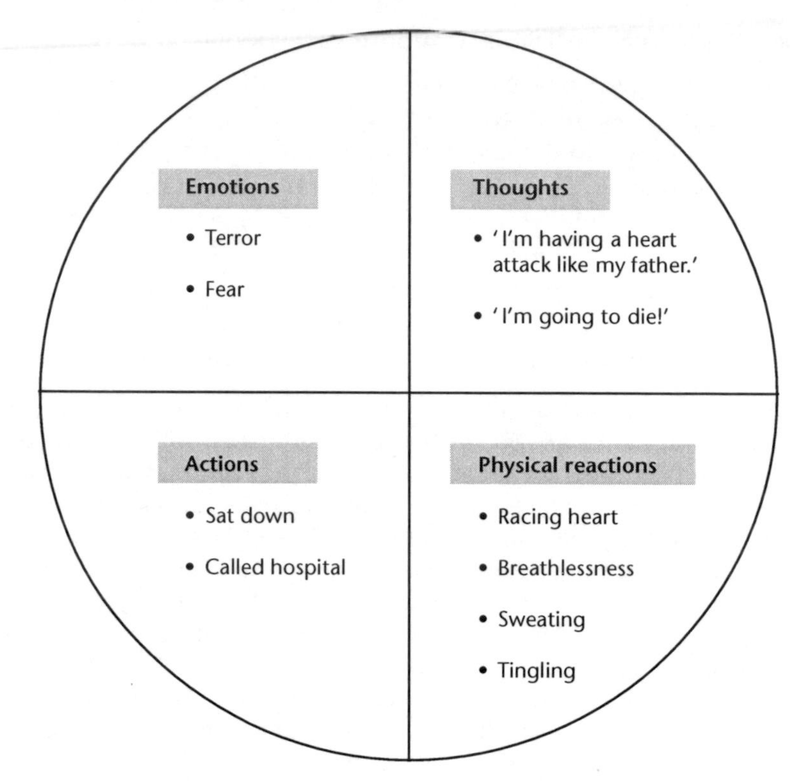

Figure 3.2 Benito's 'hot cross bun'

Modifying solutions that haven't helped

The other main focus of CBT is making sure that the ways we try to manage panic actually work. It's crucial to your success that you monitor your progress and check that the skills and techniques you decide to try from this book actually work for you.

One way of doing this is to score your level of anxiety as you work with each technique. You might want to use a scale of 0 to 10, where 0 means you feel no anxiety and 10 means you feel as anxious as you can imagine being. For example, 10 might describe the anxiety you'd feel during a panic attack. Make a note of your score before you try the technique and then regularly check it as you practise. Although it might take time, if your chosen solution is an effective one you should see your score reduce. Here's what happened to Benito:

Eventually Benito arrived home in the UK, exhausted and worried that there was something dreadfully wrong. At work the next day he spent most of his time searching the internet for information on panic attacks and heart attacks, and decided that the only way to tell the difference was via hospital tests. Over the following two weeks he had four episodes during which he became convinced that his racing heart rate was a problem and so went to hospital. Each time he was reassured when tests showed no physical problem, but his anxiety would only reduce when that had been done.

When a hospital doctor noticed that Benito had been admitted five times in under three weeks and found physically healthy each time, he suggested that he ask his GP to refer him to a psychologist for help in managing panic.

Benito had developed an understandable but anxiety-provoking, time-consuming and unhelpful way of managing his panic. His solution was to admit himself to hospital to check for medical problems. To an extent that worked: each time Benito left hospital reassured he was all right 'for now'. Every time he noticed his heart racing, however, he'd think, 'This time it really is a heart attack' and would only calm down significantly after talking to a doctor. While getting reassurance was effective, Benito's solution often involved disruption to his daily life as it needed hours in hospital up to three times a week. It also meant that he never learned any other way of coping with his symptoms of panic. Benito's understandable and seemingly logical attempts to manage his panic created significant difficulties and didn't provide a long-term solution.

While Benito's attempted solution might seem extreme, many people we work with have made huge efforts to manage their panic by applying solutions based on common sense or logic. Many whose experience of panic involves uncomfortable physical symptoms will react by sitting down, finding something to lean on or avoiding exercise or activities they enjoy in an attempt to manage those symptoms. When those symptoms subside, they associate success with those solutions and never learn that the symptoms would go away in their own time anyway. That means that they live with significant restrictions and disruption and have a solution that 'treats' but doesn't solve the problem.

Anxiety, fear and panic are unpleasant, and you'll probably have worked very hard to try to manage them. For some people that may work for a time, often years. Eventually, however, most solutions to psychological difficulties – and especially panic – based on logic will break down. That's often the point at which people come to a psychologist or therapist for help. Long-lasting solutions generally need the psychological approach we describe in this book, which is based on research and clinical experience but may sometimes not seem logical!

Even working with a psychologist, counsellor or therapist, you may not start with exactly the right solution for you. The important thing is to monitor the solutions you try and only continue using them if they work for you.

Physical symptoms and medical conditions

A large majority of the people we work with talk about the physical symptoms of panic as the overwhelming part of what they experience, and those symptoms are generally similar or even identical to those of a heart attack or other serious condition. Psychologists, counsellors and therapists aren't medically qualified and can't accurately identify medical conditions. If there's ever any doubt, you should always consult your GP or other health professional. Once underlying physical causes have been ruled out it will generally be safe to follow a psychological approach to managing those symptoms.

How what you think contributes to panic

Generally, the overwhelming feature of panic is a combination of frightening physical sensations and thoughts that focus on disastrous or catastrophic consequences of either those physical sensations or the situation that triggered your panic. Benito, for example, struggled with a racing heart rate and the conviction that he was having a heart attack. In the previous chapter, Duane was struggling with a fear of flying and Lisa with juggling life as a new mother with a stressful job. All three, and often others we work with, were caught up in a vicious cycle in which the way they thought and what they paid attention to produced feelings of panic that were maintained by what they did to keep themselves safe. We've drawn this out in Figure 3.3, using Benito's experience as an example.

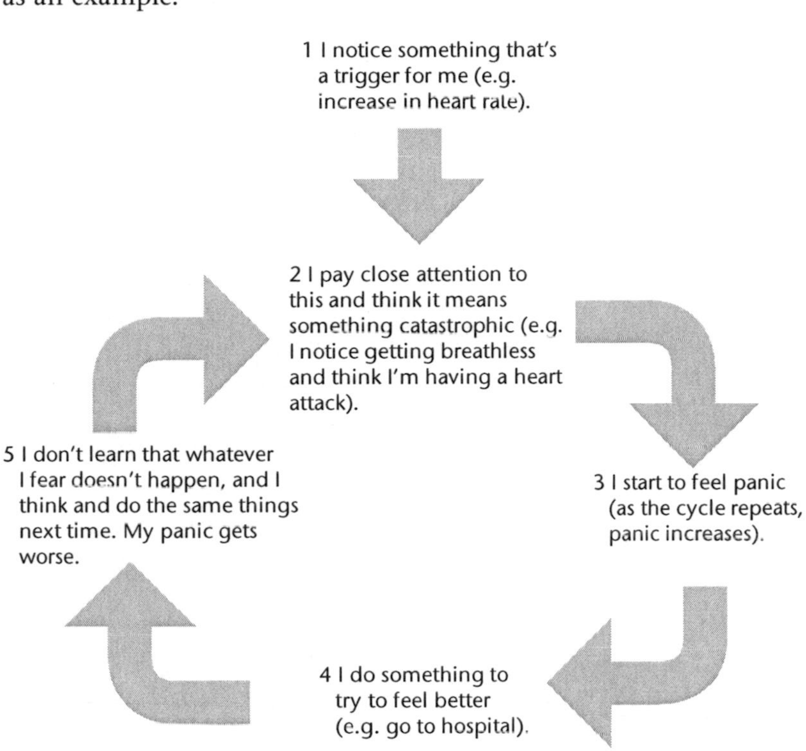

Figure 3.3 Vicious cycle of panic

Source: Based on David Westbrook, Helen Kennerley and Joan Kirk, *An Introduction to Cognitive Behaviour Therapy: Skills and Applications*, London: Sage, 2007.

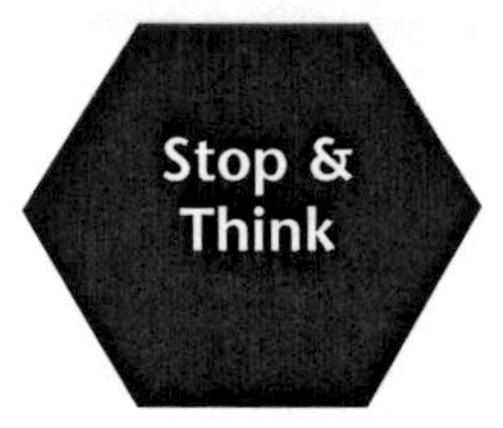

Try to draw your own vicious cycle of panic. What situations, events, physical sensations or people trigger your anxiety? What do you pay attention to in those situations? What do you do when you feel panicky? What's the result of doing that?

Most people who've had panic attacks will do their very best to manage what they think might be the catastrophic outcome. That generally involves doing two things: first, frequently or even constantly scanning for whatever triggers panic (checking your pulse, looking out for a difficult colleague at work and so on); second, assuming that the very worst will happen (for example, 'My heart is racing, so I'm having a heart attack'; 'My manager's going to give me more work and I can't cope'). As Figure 3.3 shows, thinking that way almost has to make you feel anxious or panicky, and that will make you *do* something to manage that. If what you do, such as going to hospital to get reassurance or never telling your manager that you struggle, reduces your panic, you will, understandably, probably do the same thing next time. Unfortunately, what we – seemingly logically – do may reinforce our tendency to panic in future. For example, going to hospital may be reassuring, but if there's no medical problem you'll have spent several anxious hours waiting to see a doctor and won't have learnt how to break your cycle of panic. Similarly, trying to avoid a stress-inducing manager may help you feel better for a while, but he or she will probably catch you later, by which stage you may have become even more anxious about your workload and more likely to panic.

Breaking the vicious cycle of panic almost always involves working with what you *think* and what you *do*. That's why the chapters that follow will show you how to control the three main causes of the panic cycle: what you pay attention to, what you think and what you do. We'll also describe a number of relaxation techniques aimed at directly managing the physical sensations of panic.

4

Understanding your panic

Everyone feels panicky at some time and in certain situations, but pervasive and more persistent forms of panic can provoke uncomfortable physical sensations and distressing feelings of fear. Panic attacks are common but not always a sign of serious mental health issues. They're usually accompanied by an intense fear or a sense that something awful is about to happen. There are as many different fears as there are people who panic. Some people fear that they could die or faint, others that they'll shame or make fools of themselves. Those who experience panic attacks react to bodily changes, feelings, being in certain places and memories of experiences as if they were a danger or a threat. This can be very difficult for the individual and others because it can make everyday situations feel uncomfortable and restricts and interferes with their lives. Research shows that it's often our fear and response to symptoms of panic – such as a racing heart, deep heavy breathing and sweating – that trigger the panic attack in the first place. If you have panic attacks, to understand properly how it affects you it may be time to look at how you react and cope. This chapter illustrates some of the ways panic presents, and helps you map your individual problem as a first step to selecting various techniques that will gradually help you manage attacks.

Jonathan describes a range of physical sensations and emotions during one of his panic attacks:

> I was fine until I felt a sudden sense of nausea and dizziness. When was the last time I slept? I can't remember, because the days and nights can become rather blurred when you're trying to finish an important project at work. The deadline was last week and there's no doubt that I'm super-stressed. I can feel my hands and knees shaking . . . here we go . . . I can't even type on my keyboard any more. The letters on the screen are dancing in front of me like angels . . . or is it actually ghosts I'm seeing? My vision is blurred. What's happening to me? I'm going to collapse . . .

> my breathing is getting heavier and my heart beats so fast it sounds like I've just completed the London Marathon. This doesn't feel right . . . I'm going to pass out. I grip the edge of my desk so hard my knuckles turn almost white . . . this will stop me from falling when I faint . . . I close my eyes and wait . . . and wait . . . and wait. But I don't faint and I think that I'm lucky this time around . . . I wait in anticipation for another spell of panic: sometimes it comes and sometimes it doesn't.

Jonathan's story illustrates common fears that are likely to enter or surge through your mind during a panic attack. These thoughts understandably increase anxiety and help maintain those dreadful feelings of panic. It's important to remember that most of what you fear can't or won't come true. Being prepared to examine these fears in detail and challenge the ones that aren't completely accurate is a very effective way of managing panic. Just because we think or worry that something may happen doesn't necessarily mean it's going to happen. Jonathan, for example, thought he was going to faint and gripped the edge of his desk.

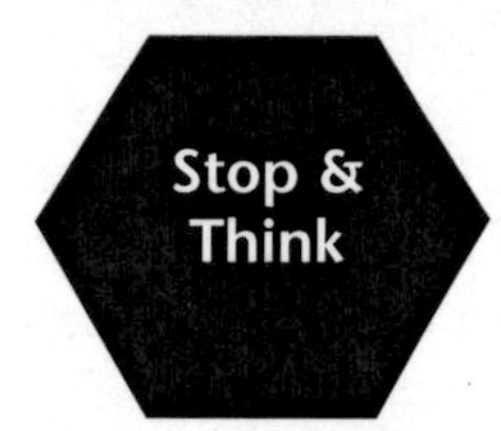

Can you think back to the last time you had a panic attack?
Did what you feared come about? What actually happened?

You may have panicked and felt out of control on a number of occasions, but that doesn't mean the catastrophe you anticipated up to and during the attack actually took place. Nevertheless, when you feel panicky these thoughts seem very intense, frightening and real. Below are some of the common thoughts people may experience during a panic attack. They're just examples, and as we said above, there are as many fears as there are people who panic.

- I'm going to have a heart attack.
- I won't be able to breathe – I'll suffocate.
- I'll be physically sick.
- I'll faint or lose consciousness.
- I'll be trapped. I'll freeze and not be able to move.
- I'm going to make a fool of myself in front of my colleagues/ friends/partner.

- I'll collapse and people will think I'm ill or mentally ill.
- I'm going to lose control – I'll be taken for a psychiatric assessment or people will think I'm weird.

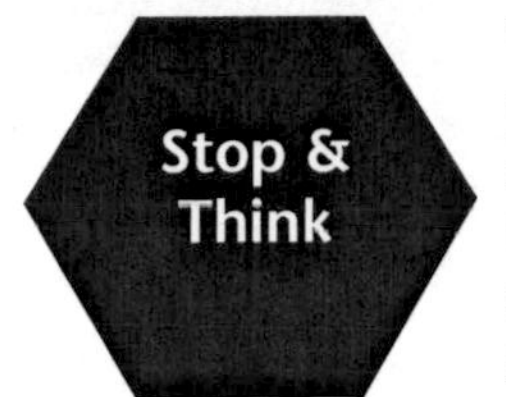

What happens to your thinking when you're panicking? What do you notice most? Can you recall any particular thoughts you're having? Take a few moments to make a note of your unique fears.

Bodily sensations

During a panic attack people usually have clearly defined bodily sensations they can describe afterwards. Just experiencing any one of them can make you feel upset, frightened or at times even desperate. Some of the physical signs of anxiety can mimic acute physical or mental illness, which can be all the more frightening and make things feel even worse.

Tracey, a 27-year-old fashion designer, suffered her first panic attack when she was 16, while waiting for a physical examination by the nurse at her local GP surgery. She recalls a tingling sensation travelling down her spine before her body felt heavy and numb. At the time she thought something was seriously wrong with her and that perhaps the headache she was also experiencing could be a symptom of a brain tumour or even a stroke. The nurse asked her to lie down and dimmed the light in the room, thinking Tracey had a migraine.

During the lead-up to her first panic attack, Tracey was feeling incredibly anxious about her impending GCSE exams. She complained about frequent stomach aches, which led her mother to book a health check with the nurse the week before her exams. Tracey experienced three more panic attacks over the next two months, each of which started with a tingling sensation. For the next 11 years she'd avoid any situation where she noticed a tingling sensation in her body. This included avoiding going to the cinema, attending a physical health examination and watching programmes that contained images of illness, such as medical soaps. She was diagnosed with irritable bowel syndrome in her early twenties and continued to worry excessively about work, relationships, finances and her family.

It was her boyfriend who encouraged her to see a therapist after

> Tracey had suffered a panic attack while at a friend's engagement party. She felt deeply embarrassed, fearing that her boyfriend and friends might think she was 'weird' or 'weak'. She felt she should be able to contain her fears and not let others see what she perceived as a weakness and flaw in her personality. Since both her parents were prone to worry and anxiety she assumed, for years, that she'd never be able to overcome her problem. Tracey attended weekly therapy sessions for the next two months, where she was gradually able to manage her worry and panic.

Psychologists treating those who have fears and panic attacks recognize that the physical symptoms can paradoxically trigger an increase in fear, which often only makes the symptoms feel worse. Tracey, for example, thought that the headache combined with the tingling sensation could indicate serious physical illness. This is what can happen when people have a panic attack. Some of their bodily sensations may be misinterpreted as indicating some kind of acute health problem.

Prolonged anxiety states can affect a person's physical health by, for example, resulting in higher and more prolonged levels of cortisol in the bloodstream. Certain physical problems may be related to psychological difficulties, and these are termed 'psychosomatic'. The most common psychosomatic problems associated with panic are over-breathing or hyperventilation, rapid heart rate, sweating and nausea. These can be managed by treating both the symptoms as well as the underlying anxiety. Some psychosomatic processes associated with anxiety and stress are dry skin and eczema, irritable bowel syndrome (IBS), blurred vision, medically unexplained headaches and digestive problems.

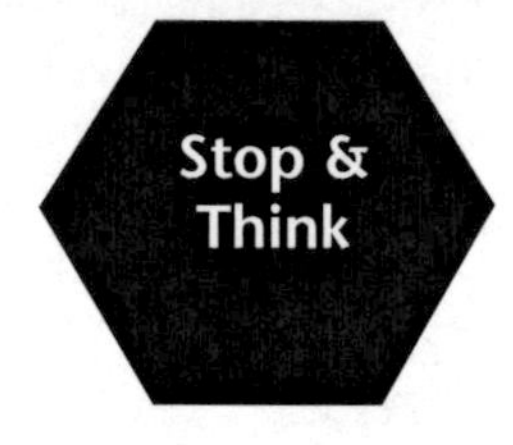

How does your body react when you're stressed? What do you notice most? What are the most unpleasant sensations for you? Take a few moments to make a note of your unique reactions.

Actions or behaviours

When something as frightening as a panic attack occurs, you may try to do something to prevent the harm that seems to threaten you. When the fear is intense enough, our animal-like instincts take over. This will often cause a person to respond to critical events in one of three ways, or a combination of them, known as fight–flight–freeze responses. You may, for example, try to escape from the situation you're in so that you can reach a physically or emotionally safer place. Another common way that people behave when they panic is to try to avoid similar situations in future:

> Mustafa, a man in his late 50s, was waiting to pay for his shopping at his local supermarket when he experienced several upsetting symptoms, including tightness in the throat, breathlessness and shakiness, together with a fear of suffocation. He put his shopping basket down and left, returning home as quickly as possible. He remained frightened and exhausted for days after the event. His GP couldn't find any physical origin for his symptoms, and suggested Mustafa may have had a panic attack. Mustafa was so terrified of another attack that he stopped going out to do his shopping. He was also worried that his colleagues might witness him having another panic attack while at work, and perhaps think that he was mad. He started to work more from home and became increasingly reluctant to leave the house. He was well on the way to developing agoraphobia when he came to see us.

As you can see from this example, Mustafa wanted to get out of the supermarket so that he could go home where he felt safer. This is the 'flight' response being activated. He then began to avoid going to the supermarket and going to work, which eventually led him to stay at home much of the time. This problem is termed agoraphobia.

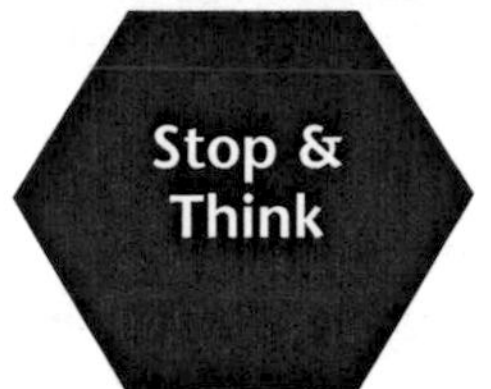

Try to identify your own panic-related behaviours. Is there anything in particular that you do when you feel panicky? Do you avoid situations that are anxiety provoking or do you confront them? Are your actions helpful or unhelpful?

As you read on you'll learn more about how your actions and behaviours may sometimes maintain your panic, and how to replace unhelpful behaviours with more helpful ones.

Panic and fear

In terms of psychological difficulties, fears and panic are both similar to and in some ways different from other problems such as low mood (depression), obsessive–compulsive disorder or having an eating problem. Here are some ideas on what's unique and specific about experiencing panic attacks and fears.

- The effects are usually intense and can in some cases require psychological and medical intervention.
- They're often triggered by some form of pressure, fear, unpleasant sensations and feelings, stress, worry, health concerns or over-exertion; the signs and symptoms can come out of the blue or onset can be gradual.
- Often both the mind and the body are affected, possibly making us feel out of control and overwhelmed, which in turn increases our anxiety. This effect could produce such physical symptoms as, among others, hyperventilation, a sense of choking, increased heart rate, dizziness.

Panic attacks can arise in certain situations but not in others. They're unpleasant and typically lead to withdrawal from situations that we fear may have triggered them. This is because we come to learn that our anxiety and physical sensations may increase if we have to deal with these situations again. Avoidance ultimately only makes the fear worse because we quickly build up a defensive story about why we can't attend a party, go shopping or do something else that involves standing up to our fear. Life may then become a series of rituals designed to make us feel safer, and may be dominated by attempts at avoidance. The problem with this behaviour is that it prevents exposure, which in turn can thwart the opportunity to build the confidence we need to manage our panic. Some methods of coping reflect understandable but unhealthy approaches, such as making excuses to bow out of commitments or excessive use of alcohol to help quell one's nerves during a work lunch or when travelling by air. These actions are easily available remedies to dampen down the panic, but they don't offer a longer-lasting solution to overcoming it. When the short-term effects wear off, we often experience greater anxiety again.

Exploring your own experience of panic

One way to understand your own experience of panic better is to ask yourself whether you feel frightened across a wide range of situations or rather in relation to more specific things, such as certain people, places, feelings, experiences or events.

Sometimes the panic attacks seem to go on and on, and fear of a fear can become a lifelong problem if left untreated. There can be a number of reasons for this. Some people may have an anxious personality or have 'learnt' to worry. Others may have experienced stressful life events such as bereavement, redundancy or relationship problems. Others may be under pressure at work, or at home because of family problems or financial difficulties.

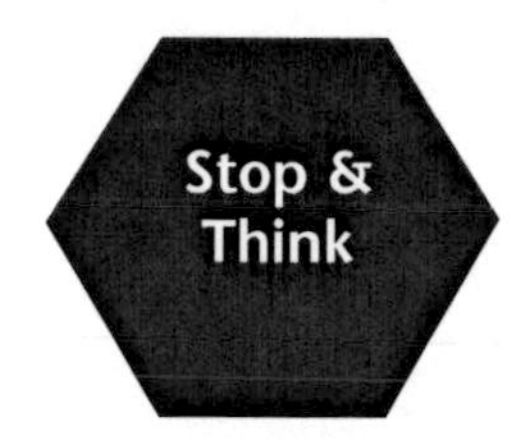

How often do you feel panicky? (Often, rarely, sometimes, never?) What kinds of situations are most likely to make you feel frightened, anxious or panicky? (Meeting new people, travelling, completing work projects, going on a date, being in crowded places, financial/health or relationship concerns?) How long do your panic attacks last? (Seconds, minutes?) Is there a pattern to your panic? (Does it occur on a specific day, in a specific context/place or with particular people?) How does it affect your eating, sleeping, concentration, memory, sex drive, energy, motivation and so on?

It's important to recognize that each person's experience of panic attacks is unique: what's perceived as anxiety provoking by one person may not be by another. This can be reassuring in itself, and means we might be able to ask: 'Why do other people seem to cope better in these situations?' Now that you've reached this stage in the book you'll have begun to realize that we all react to stressful and anxiety-provoking situations in different ways. Your best friend, for example, might be very confident in challenging situations that tend to make you feel anxious, but terrified of going to the dentist! The manager you admire for her skill and confidence in charming new clients may just naturally be that way, or maybe she's just very good at concealing her anxiety. In either case, you may find it helpful to ask them for hints on how they cope in stressful situations – or even to copy how they react to them.

5

Why haven't I overcome my panic attacks?

Some people we've helped have asked: 'What drives or maintains my panic attacks?' This is a good question and the answer may be reassuring and helpful to some readers. Anxiety problems usually come from a distorted belief about the level of danger associated with certain situations, bodily sensations or mental events. Once we've experienced anxious feelings, the same or similar situations, feelings and bodily and mental sensations can reactivate fear and anxiety. Nobody likes feelings of anxiety or panic, and you've probably worked hard to find ways to reduce yours. Unfortunately, solutions based only on common sense or logic are often effective just in the short term and may even help maintain panic attacks. This chapter will show you alternative strategies for managing your panic attacks based on the psychological approach we described in Chapter 3. Imagine that you were fearful of having confrontations with work colleagues or friends. If you continued to avoid speaking your mind or were too afraid to verbalize what you felt needed to be said, it's likely that the problem of dreading confrontations would persist. An effective solution might be to learn how gradually to be more forthcoming with your opinions – this could eventually stop you from keeping silent when you disagree with other people's views.

Panic is one of many psychological problems that require the right key to fit the lock. It also requires time, persistence and patience to achieve satisfactory outcomes. We're optimistic that almost everyone can learn to manage panic attacks. Christina, for example, was able to overcome hers with the help of her psychologist:

> I never thought I'd be able to overcome my panic. I attended two different courses on how to beat panic attacks and live a more fulfilling life. I survived the compulsory trip to the supermarket with the group

facilitator holding my hand, but I couldn't get myself to do it on my own. I eventually sought help from a psychologist. He was very helpful and taught me how to challenge unhelpful thoughts. I became a master at relaxation skills and I started to do some things differently. I used to think that my 'safety behaviours' were effective ways of keeping me safe. It was a difficult journey but one that changed my life for ever. I think my family and friends were shocked when I started to attend social events again. I still get apprehensive about crowded places but I'm no longer terrified.

Unhelpful coping strategies

How can you break free from the vicious cycle of panic? It may feel like your panic attacks can go on and on despite your best efforts to try to overcome them. You may have already tried coping techniques, none of which have worked and some of which may reflect understandable but unhelpful approaches. In particular, while they may quell anxiety for a short time, for some people their use simply masks the problem or may even worsen the effects of anxiety.

Psychologists working with people who have anxiety have recently turned their attention to what maintains panic attacks as much as to what causes them. Some common factors – unhelpful strategies – can keep you having attacks, and it's important to recognize these and understand how they might affect you.

Avoidance

You may avoid situations, people or places that you fear may cause another panic attack. It's perfectly normal to try to avoid something that you think is dangerous, but if the situation is safe it may be more your fears that prevent you from staying around and finding out that the danger may not be real. If, for example, you avoid going to crowded places at all times, you may never discover that you won't faint, have a heart attack, be sick in front of people or whatever else you may fear. In many cases, avoidance can make panic worse because it keeps you from realizing that you can cope with situations you fear. It can also result in a great loss of confidence, which can affect how you feel about yourself.

Over-reliance on trying to stay safe

Panic and anxiety can drive us to behave in ways that we think will help us feel safe, or at least less anxious. These actions may not be helpful in the long run because they act in various ways to keep you believing there's a real danger. Paul, for example, only went to the supermarket when he was with someone else with whom he felt safe. The problem was that he never got the chance to find out that no harm would come to him even if he went shopping by himself. He thought having someone with him prevented him from fainting or having another panic attack. Doing this meant Paul could never find out that he was actually unlikely to faint in the supermarket. Other common safety behaviours include carrying a paper bag in case you're sick; resting or avoiding exercise to prevent you from having a heart attack; holding on to something like a lamppost or a chair to prevent you from collapsing; lying down and raising your feet in the air to reduce the chance of fainting; always attempting to sit close to an exit so that you can escape more easily if you 'need' to.

Trying to predict the future

Another challenge for people who have panic attacks is that they often start to fear situations where they've previously experienced panic and anxiety. They're afraid that another attack may occur and sometimes the fear is so strong that it can trigger physical symptoms of anxiety. As we mentioned in Chapter 2, this is known as anticipatory anxiety. A vicious cycle often occurs where previous panic attacks lead to negative thoughts such as 'What if I have another panic attack? No one will help me; they may think I'm mad.' This in turn reinforces the dread of being in a situation where panic has occurred, which could mean you become too scared to stay in a fear-inducing situation to see what happens.

Focusing too much on bodily sensations

A person who's experienced a panic attack in the past may 'scan' his or her body several times for signs of a pending panic attack. This is to be vigilant to the possibility that they may feel ill, have a panic attack or lose bodily control (fainting, vomiting, over-breathing and so on). If you're checking your body too much you may risk mistaking normal bodily changes for physical symptoms of panic. A good example is when a person misinterprets normal changes in their breathing following exercise or physical exertion as signs of breathing difficulties or even suffocation. The more a person checks, the more uncertain they'll feel, and that often helps maintain panic and anxiety.

Catastrophic interpretation of symptoms

The physical sensations of panic can feel similar to the symptoms of physiological events. For example, people who struggle with panic may become very frightened if they notice their heart rate has increased, because they think it could mean they're having a heart attack. In fact many people experience minor changes in their heart rate when they enter less familiar situations, such as sitting an important exam or meeting prospective parents-in-law – neither of which they're likely to do every day. The body recognizes the newness or unfamiliarity of the situation and prepares us to react in order to cope. These normal bodily signs or reactions can lead some people to believe, mistakenly, that there's something mentally or physically wrong with them, and they can become very frightened. Once any actual medical causes have been checked for, learning to think of the rapid heart rate and feeling faint – in this example – as symptoms of anxiety that can be controlled can significantly reduce anxiety.

Being selective of what we pay attention to

A further point to notice is that our memory is selective and may confirm our worst nightmare scenario, even if there's only a small possibility that the worst is happening. We may fixate on the negative aspect of an experience. For example, we might have felt overwhelmed by our anxiety and suffered a panic attack. However unpleasant this might have been, it's likely we recovered from this and eventually coped. Unfortunately, we've continued to worry about both our fear of having another panic attack as well as our extreme reaction to it. These memories are carefully stored and highlight the negative aspects of panic and how we were affected. So if you had a panic attack that lasted five minutes but you coped well for the rest of the time, learning to increase your focus on the amount of time you coped could reduce your anxiety.

Excessive worry

If you're spending too much time concentrating on your panic, you may be reinforcing your fear and reducing your capacity to do anything constructive to manage it. You may think that by worrying about feared events you will be able to prevent them happening. For example, you may imagine a number of catastrophic events prior to and during a panic-inducing situation and make a mental note on how to deal with each of them. Often these anticipated disasters may be products of our imagined worries rather than probable events, but allowing yourself to focus on these worries can significantly increase your anxiety.

Excessive use of alcohol or recreational drugs

Some people may use alcohol to help them quell their nerves when they're feeling anxious or panicky. However, anxiety often re-emerges soon after as the effect of the alcohol wears off, and they may end up with the added problems of dehydration and a hangover. In addition, they have the potential to develop a new problem: over-reliance on alcohol. This can lead them to attribute their ability to stay in a panic-inducing situation to its use rather than other skills and techniques. Alcohol may seem a useful and easily available remedy to anxiety, but it doesn't help you overcome it. Very occasionally, even prescribed medications can have the same unwanted effect, so it's always advisable to check with your GP whether medications you may be on can increase stress and anxiety.

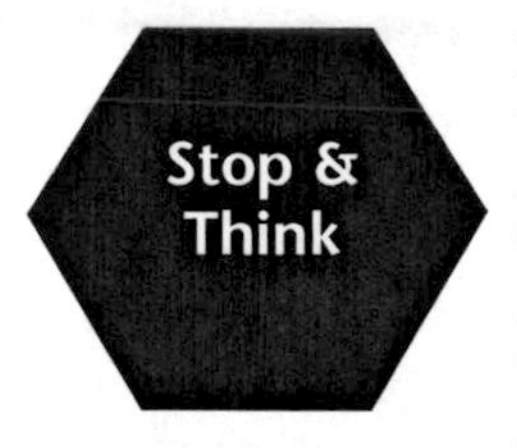

Note some of the things you've done or would do to make yourself feel safe during a situation you fear. Make a distinction between ordinary safety precautions (using a seat belt while driving) and safety behaviours that prevent you from relaxing (being overly aware of physical sensations, worrying excessively about having another panic attack). Select one safety behaviour you might like to stop – to reduce anxiety, you need to reduce these behaviours. This is best done by focusing on each safety behaviour in turn. Ask yourself: 'Is my feared disaster likely to occur if I stop [the specific action you're doing]?' 'Will I feel more relaxed and comfortable if I stop [the specific action you're doing]?'

Below you'll find a list of the more common explanations of why you continue to experience difficulty with panic. This is by no means exhaustive, but it will serve as a checklist against which you can measure your own progress and ongoing difficulties. If you have some grasp of why you continue to struggle with your problem, you should gain a deeper awareness of how it affects you and how modern psychological theory helps us understand how different people progress at different rates in their treatment.

Some reasons why progress may be slow

If, for example, your attempted solution to panic is to avoid confronting situations you feel may be causing symptoms of panic, this is unlikely to help you make much progress. There's a wide range of cognitive and behavioural techniques, skills and interventions that you can use to challenge and overcome panic. However, if you stay away from situations where you can test out their effectiveness or measure your progress, then they're merely textbook ideas. At some point we need to move the ideas from the page or the laboratory into the real world and test how they work for us. This can sometimes be daunting, stressful or even feel emotionally too painful. If this is the case, we may need to go back a step or two so that we're not overwhelmed by our feelings. With most psychological difficulties, it's preferable to take gradual, comfortable but determined steps forward and to gain confidence, rather than giant leaps and risk all. There's little point in escalating stress and anxiety to levels that feel too uncomfortable or even unbearable. It may be necessary to try something different or less difficult. For example, if one attempted solution to your problem was to try to attend a work function you feared, but you'd had to leave the party early feeling significantly more stressed than before you set out, then perhaps you attempted too big a first step. It may be worth scaling your next intervention back to attending a small gathering in your local coffee shop with close friends and family.

So gaining confidence via these small steps is arguably better than taking giant leaps that would expose you to greater stress and anxiety, and potentially put you off overcoming your difficulty. In addition, if your thoughts about what you need to do leave you feeling emotionally vulnerable and upset, then it's perhaps time to go back to gaining a clearer understanding of them and to explore your fundamental fear about what it is you think could happen to you. It may be that your underlying fear of some catastrophic outcome – such as having a panic attack, fainting, losing control or having a heart attack – is driving the problem. This may need further exploration and understanding, as well as targeted interventions, and such feelings can sometimes best be dealt with by speaking to a qualified specialist, such as a psychologist, counsellor or therapist.

Having the resources to put these skills into practice

Motivational issues can also interfere with progress in psychological therapy generally. This isn't to suggest that people who have psychological challenges or issues don't wish to overcome them – most of the time this isn't the case. However, we may not always give the time, focus and intensity needed to overcome the problem sufficiently. This may be because we're stressed or facing other difficulties in our lives that distract us from dealing with the problem in hand. Very few people have the luxury of working on their panic without having other issues to deal with. It may be that we're having a difficult time at work, for example, are stressed by a child or facing health problems in the family. Motivation may also be affected by the simple fact that we've lived with the problem for a long time – we may have coped to the extent that we've found ways to avoid or manage rather than solve it. Sometimes being comfortable with our own solution to the problem, even though it's not a total solution, may interfere with efforts really to overcome and cure it.

Anxiety and panic require some effort if we're to overcome them. This is no different from gaining new skills in other areas of our lives. Do you remember the first time you learned how to use a computer? Probably you were one of the many people who struggled to find the on/off button, accidentally deleted documents or got stuck transferring files from one folder to another. In psychological therapy, the initial stages can feel awkward, stressful and difficult to deal with. If you're struggling with making progress, it may be helpful to reflect on and consider your motivation to overcome the problem.

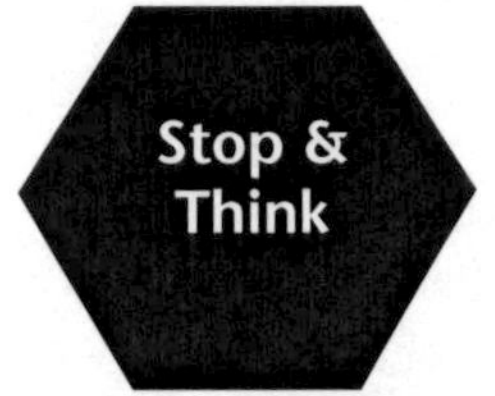

You might ask yourself a series of reflective questions to assess your circumstances and motivation, such as: 'Am I comfortable in my ways?' 'Is it too much effort to make the necessary change?' 'Do I have the energy, stamina or motivation to overcome this difficulty?' 'Are the gains I could make outweighed by the comfort I feel staying as I am?' 'Could anything else in my life be holding me back from making changes in my behaviour and dealing with uncomfortable and/or stressful feelings?'

If the solution you're using isn't helping you achieve the outcome you want, it's unlikely to be the right solution for you at this point. If, for example, you keep challenging your negative automatic thoughts about panic-inducing situations but fail to back this up with behavioural changes, your progress may be limited or temporary. Conversely, if you change some of your behaviour without considering changes to some of your thoughts about experiencing panic attacks, you may not reach your goals. For example, if you avoid going to crowded places, you may try to reduce your anxiety by standing close to the emergency exit when going to a concert. You may feel that positioning yourself close to an exit will help you cope better with the stress of the situation. However, this can easily become a safety behaviour – as many readers will know, it can inadvertently lead to over-reliance on certain conditions without which you may not be able to go to crowded places. It seems an easy solution to the problem and may initially help you confront your fear, but it's potentially a self-defeating one if you continue to rely on being able to stand next to an emergency exit every time you're in a crowded place.

Psychological problems rarely exist in total isolation from other issues going on in our lives. For example, if you're experiencing low mood, low self-esteem or have a physical health issue that affects your behaviour, these may directly affect your confidence and your feelings about being able to cope with the situations you fear. Addressing panic without taking into account these additional issues or factors may limit your progress. That's not to say that if you suffer from low self-esteem you need be completely free of any symptoms, or if from depression you should be in perfect psychological shape before addressing panic. It does mean, however, that you need to take these additional factors into account when coming to understand your panic. Again, a qualified psychologist, therapist or counsellor can provide additional help.

Setting your sights on an instant and total cure to the problem of panic is understandable but may pose too great a challenge. Experience tells us that the treatment of many fears and phobias can take time, and progress may be gradual and incremental. If you follow the psychological method of cognitive behavioural therapy that underlies this book, you can expect progress to be gradual, sometimes a bit slow, but nonetheless you should see general positive progress. Treatment, whether with a psychologist or through self-help, requires time, patience, perseverance and a great deal of determination. There may be occasional setbacks or at times it may feel as if you're playing a game of Snakes and Ladders: as if progress has been suddenly reversed, but just as quickly picks up again. Maintaining a positive outlook, a healthy dose of motivation, and keeping the ideas described in this book in mind, will help keep you focused and on track.

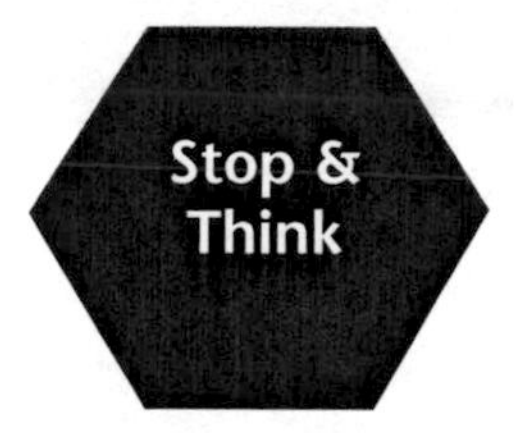

Is your goal realistic (not too difficult but not too easy either)? Is it possible to break it into a smaller set of sub-goals? Can you think about ways to measure your progress (what you can do now that you couldn't when you started work on your goal)? Have you allowed yourself enough time to achieve your goal or goals?

Involving others – specialists – in your treatment and problem solving can be enormously helpful. However, it may be that the act of describing the problem to someone else is the first and most obvious stumbling block. Perhaps it would be embarrassing or stressful even to describe the problem to another person. Also, bringing oneself into close emotional proximity to others is something many people find difficult. We would encourage you to do this because, in our experience, trained and experienced specialists in this area will have encountered many people with similar problems before. For them, this won't be new and nor will it be an uncomfortable situation. On the contrary, it's their job to help you with this difficulty, and they should give you every encouragement along the way. Given that it's a treatable psychological condition, you can expect support and help in your efforts to overcome it. Your starting point, if you take the problem to a trained specialist, could be that you've recently read a book on overcoming panic (this one!) and, on the basis of what you've read, you think you might have this condition. If you've been able to apply some of the ideas you've learnt in the book, you may also be able to describe why and how you feel the problem has come about and what you've done so far to overcome it. You could also possibly describe why you feel you're not making adequate progress in overcoming it. We recognize that taking the problem to someone else means facing up to it and verbalizing it to another person. Think of it as part of your therapy in that describing the problem and talking about it with another is in itself therapeutic. Describing our problems is a major way in which we learn more about how they affect us and how we feel about them. It's an important next step in bringing about change.

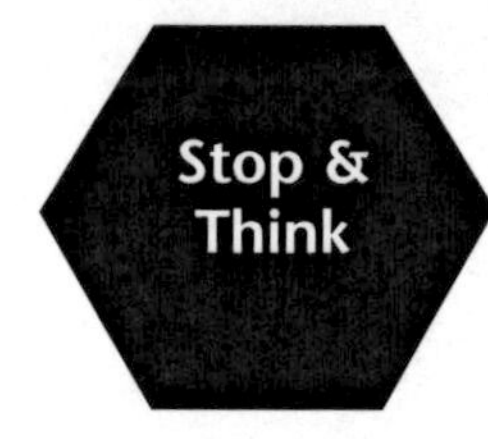

Is there anyone you can think of who you might find it easier to talk to (a friend, family member, colleague or teacher)? When would be the best time for you to talk to others about the issues you're experiencing? What would you essentially want the other person to do (just listen, offer practical advice on how best to manage your panic, offer empathy and understanding, help you find a psychologist, therapist or counsellor)?

A session with your GP, psychologist, counsellor or therapist will help put you back on track by assessing the nature and extent of your problem and how best to treat it. This book can then act as a companion to that face-to-face treatment. You can use it to help you think about homework exercises and in plotting your progress in overcoming panic. The next chapter will take you through the ways in which what you do can help manage your panic.

6

Managing panic

By now you'll have realized that managing panic requires working with what you do and what you think (and as the next chapter will discuss, it also requires learning to manage physical symptoms using relaxation skills). New ways of doing things can often be a really effective way of breaking into your unique cycle of panic. This chapter looks at practical ways of trying out new behaviours and building your confidence in order to overcome your panic. Cognitive behavioural therapy (CBT) offers some ways of working with what you do to produce a more effective solution. We'll start by describing how to select and try the solutions most likely to be effective for you, and then describe the techniques most likely to be effective in overcoming panic.

Is this technique working for me?

Using the information you've collected as you worked through the earlier chapters, you'll have a good chance of choosing a technique that's likely to be effective for you. Nobody, however, and certainly not psychologists, gets it right first time every time. That why it's so important to monitor the techniques you select and not invest too much time and effort in trying to make a solution work if it isn't effective for you.

When you've selected a technique from this book to help manage your individual panic, start by reading the description of that technique again and make sure you understand why you've chosen to try it, why it may be helpful for you and what it involves. As we said earlier, sharing some of the work you're doing with a trusted friend or relative can be enormously helpful. If you have someone helping you, a good way of checking that you understand the technique is to try to explain to them what it is and why you're doing it. If you can do that, you can be confident that you understand what you're doing – and if you find it difficult, they may be able to help.

Once you understand what you're trying to achieve, it's equally important to be sure how you'll know you've used an effective solution for you. How you measure that will depend on exactly what you're doing and what you're aiming to achieve.

Here are some suggested ways you could monitor your progress.

- Give your feeling of anxiety or panic a score of 0 to 10, where 0 is feeling perfectly calm and 10 refers to maximum panic. When you're in situations that have triggered panic for you in the past, make a note of your score. If the techniques you're using are effective, your score will reduce with practice. This type of monitoring is especially useful if you're using the 'graded exposure' techniques we describe shortly.
- Alternatively, you could ask a trusted friend or relative to score how anxious you appear. This can be a really useful confidence boost if you tend to panic in situations where you worry about what other people think of you.
- Count the number of times you do things that either help manage your panic or contribute to it. If the technique is working for you, unhelpful behaviours will reduce and helpful ones will increase.
- Set a sensible goal and plan a reward for when you achieve it. There's a brief section on how to create goals later in this chapter.

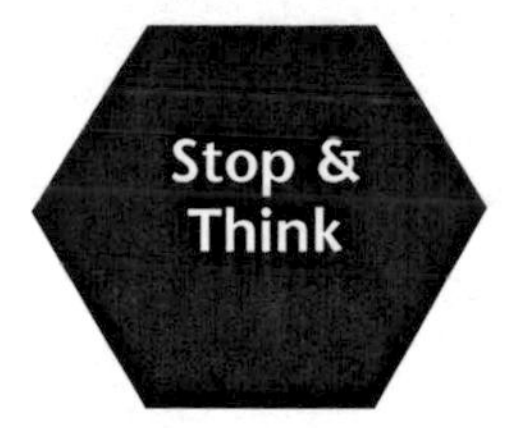

When you've selected a technique you'd like to try, come back to the list of ways to monitor progress and think about how you'll monitor yours. You might like to use a notebook so you can see how far you've come. How will you know you're making progress? What's your goal in using that technique?

Changing 'logical' solutions that aren't working

You now know that the most obvious solutions based on common sense may not be effective in overcoming panic in the long term. Psychologists call these 'safety behaviours' because they're what you do to try to keep yourself safe. You'll have come to realize that to manage your panic effectively, it may be necessary to change or even stop doing these things. Here's how Emily managed to stop her safety behaviour:

> Following an accident on a motorway, Emily would only drive on local roads unless her husband was with her. On her own she'd become increasingly anxious driving on the motorway and full-blown panic would set in rapidly. When her sister, who lived over two hours away by motorway, became seriously ill, Emily needed to be able to drive on the motorway without her husband. She asked her GP to refer her to a counsellor for help.
>
> Emily and her counsellor identified needing her husband to be with her as a safety behaviour. It had previously been an effective way of helping Emily feel safe on the motorway as her husband was very calm as a passenger in the car and would often point out how safely she was driving. With her sister ill, however, Emily needed to be able to cope without him.
>
> Emily and her counsellor talked about why she felt calmer when her husband was in the car and identified a number of factors. As well as being a calming influence, Emily thought of him as an extra pair of eyes. This was particularly reassuring for her as her accident had been caused by a car changing lanes in her 'blind spot' when she'd been driving alone. Using some of the techniques in Chapter 9, they started to challenge those thoughts, and Emily came to see that she was a genuinely safe driver and the accident wouldn't have been prevented had her husband been there.
>
> To reinforce this new way of thinking, Emily took an advanced driver's course to boost her confidence, and with her counsellor's encouragement began to take short journeys on the motorway alone. She was delighted to discover that she could now control her anxiety. Eventually she was able to drive to her sister's home without any panic attacks. Emily found that she quickly gained confidence once she stopped relying on her safety behaviour.

It's important to understand why a solution you may have worked very hard to implement isn't being effective. For most people we've worked with it's vital to replace that solution with one that provides a long-term answer. For Emily that meant improving her confidence with training and working with what she thought before driving on her own. For others it might mean changing what they do gradually, trying out new ways of doing something or reducing a behaviour that may not be helpful in the long term. Often these techniques need to be combined with learning to relax and working with what you think, as we describe in Chapters 7, 8 and 9. The remainder of this chapter focuses on those 'doing' techniques.

Learning not to avoid things that are genuinely safe – 'graded exposure'

One of the most common things we see people do to try to manage anxiety of any kind is to avoid whatever provokes that anxiety. As we showed you earlier, however, there are many reasons why doing this may not be an effective solution and may have unacceptable consequences. If you've started to realize that you might be doing this and whatever you're avoiding is safe, learning to sit through anxiety-provoking situations is a vital tool in managing your panic. Psychologists call the technique we describe here 'graded exposure'. Essentially it involves working towards being in contact with whatever makes you anxious ('exposure') in progressive ('graded') steps that are challenging but achievable.

Graded exposure means following these steps:

1. Define what you're trying to do – your goal – and estimate how anxious that will make you feel on a scale of 0 to 10.
2. Make a note of what you can already do that's nearest to achieving that goal. This is your starting point.
3. Create several steps between your starting point and your goal – most people use 4 to 8 but we've worked with some who needed 15 or more.
4. Start by practising the first step and rate your anxiety each time you do. Repeat that step until your anxiety reduces to an acceptable level.
5. Repeat that for each step until you achieve your goal.

6 Make sure you reward yourself for achieving your goal, and ideally for each step you complete.

Here's an example to illustrate putting these steps into practice:

Brian was confident in doing almost anything except going to the dentist. As a child his sister had teased him about the frightening and painful instruments and needles in their dentist's surgery. As soon as he left home, Brian stopped attending regular dental appointments until he was forced to seek help for a painful abscess. He had a panic attack in reception and again in the dentist's chair. Fortunately the dentist was able to do just enough to confidently prescribe antibiotics, but told Brian he'd need to return for further appointments. Brian sought advice from his GP, who recommended a psychologist.

With his psychologist, Brian set a goal of being able to attend a dental appointment of up to 30 minutes without having a panic attack and with his anxiety not increasing above 7 out of 10. They broke this down into the hierarchy of steps in Table 6.1.

Table 6.1 Brian's steps for graded exposure

Step	*Description*	*Predicted anxiety*
1	Make an appointment by telephone	5/10
2	Sit in reception without going into the treatment room	6/10
3	Sit in the dentist's chair without having treatment and with no instruments in view	7/10
4	Sit in the dentist's chair without having treatment but with instruments in view	8/10
5	Have treatment not exceeding 15 minutes	9/10
6	Have treatment for up to 30 minutes	10/10

Brian's dentist took an interest in his nervous patients and was happy to allow him to work through each of these steps several times. With his psychologist, Brian learned relaxation techniques and how to challenge the unhelpful anxious thoughts resulting from his sister's teasing. They agreed that Brian could confidently cope with an anxiety that reached 5 out of 10 and that he'd work through each step until that was achieved. Brian started by sitting in reception for 20 minutes until he could confidently reduce his anxiety, and then progressed to sitting in his dentist's chair. Eventually he'd received the treatment he needed and was able to attend regular checkups without any panic attacks.

Brian's story shows how effective working towards a goal in small manageable steps can be. The key to making this work is having a good 'fear hierarchy' or set of steps like those in Table 6.1. It's well worth taking the time to plan this out in detail. If you're finding that difficult, you might find it helpful to ask someone you trust to help. The following ideas might also be useful.

- Make sure that your final goal is 'SMART' – see the section later in this chapter.
- If it's difficult to think of a manageable step, can you add something or someone to support you the first few times you try? For example, it can be difficult to work towards getting on an aeroplane in small steps, but you might be more confident with a trusted friend or relative to start with. In this situation you might start with a short flight with a companion, then a short flight on your own. You could then build up to longer flights with and without a companion.
- Normally more than one aspect of events, objects or people triggers anxiety. You may be able to build up one aspect at a time. For example, if you almost always have panic attacks on the Underground, you might start by building confidence on short journeys that begin from overland stations, before increasing the length of the journey and time underground. You could then progress to starting and finishing at underground stations. If you panic in lifts, you might notice that your anxiety is much worse in small, dark lifts than large, open ones. Graded exposure for this situation might start with practising relaxation techniques in a large glass lift in your local shopping centre, before moving to one in, say, a local car park that's large and well lit but with solid sides. Eventually you should be able to use smaller, darker lifts confidently and without panic.

Reducing safety behaviours

If you've tried ways of overcoming panic and anxiety that haven't worked in the long term, you probably need to do something differently. Reducing safety behaviours is often the first step towards a more effective solution. As psychologists, however, we know that whatever you're currently doing started because it seemed the sensible way to manage your anxiety then, and may have been helpful in the short term. That means it's important to work towards changing what you do in a gentle and systematic way. The starting point is to be specific about what you're currently doing. Safety behaviours generally fall into one of three categories:

1 Avoiding people, events, places or objects that trigger your anxiety and panic. This is what Emily was doing when she stopped driving on the motorway.
2 Rituals or behaviours designed to keep you safe. Benito used this sort of safety behaviour when he frequently went to hospital (see Chapter 3).
3 Only doing certain things in certain conditions. Emily, for example, would initially only drive on the motorway with her husband. While this was a useful step in building her confidence, it restricted what she could do in the longer term.

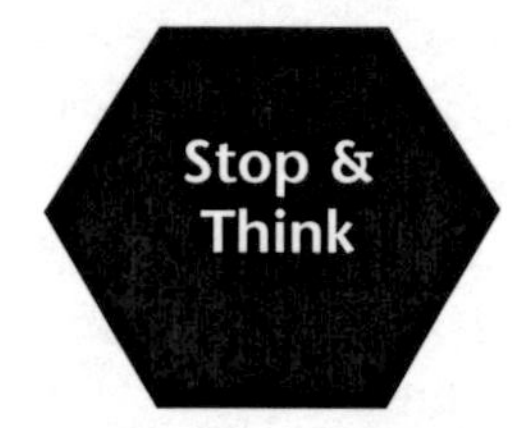

Have you identified any of your own solutions that may actually now be less effective than you'd hoped? Which of the categories above do they fall into? Can you begin to see how you might change what you do?

Using graded exposure is often a good approach to working with safety behaviour that centres on avoiding something. It can also, as Emily's experience shows, be helpful in reducing the extent to which you rely on support to do the things that make you anxious. In her case she'd come to rely on her husband, but the same approach would work for people who relied on being in a particular place or needed a special object with them to counter their anxiety.

It's unrealistic to expect to stop doing something you've found helpful without replacing that with something that effectively manages your anxiety before it becomes panic. Learning to relax is often an effective substitute. Finding a distraction may also be effective. We've worked with people who've found that focusing on a crossword puzzle or book can distract them from wanting to fall back on the solution they previously relied on. Other people have used music, yoga, exercise or finding someone to talk nonsense with! It's important to take the time to think about what might work for you, and remember that you might not find the perfect solution at your first attempt. If your initial idea doesn't work, try another way of doing things.

Noticing that what we do can change what we think

One of the reasons CBT is so effective is that what you do can often challenge unhelpful ways of thinking. Graded exposure, for example, works in two ways: first by gradually changing what you do, and second by building your confidence so that your thinking becomes less anxious. Brian's fear hierarchy was effective because at each stage he learned that the anxious thoughts he had about being at the dentist were not accurate. What he *did* changed what he *thought*. Chapters 8 and 9 have more advice on working with what you think.

Setting SMART goals

As we've already said, setting goals can be an important and useful contribution to making the techniques in this chapter work for you. If, however, you set yourself a goal that's either too difficult or too hard to know whether you've achieved it, it can add to your difficulties. Goals need to be **s**pecific, **m**easurable, **a**chievable, **r**ealistic and **t**ime-limited – SMART.

Specific If you can describe your goal in a way that defines exactly what it is, you're more likely to be able to see your progress and know when you've achieved it. 'I want to panic less' isn't specific and could be demoralizing to work towards – you're unlikely to know when you achieve it. 'I want to stop having panic attacks in team meetings' would be a specific goal.

Measurable You need to be able to measure what you're trying to achieve, or again you won't be able to see your progress. For example, 'I want to feel less anxious' can't be measured, whereas, 'I want to reduce my feeling of panic from 9/10 to 4/10 when I walk past a barking dog' is specific *and* measureable.

Achievable Make sure your goal is something you're able to achieve. For most people, 'I want to climb Everest to prove I won't panic from a fear of heights' isn't achievable, and is unlikely to be more effective than, 'I want to be able to take my grandchildren to the top of the church tower without having a panic attack'.

Realistic Make sure your goal is realistic given your physical abilities, practical resources and time. If your panic is related to a fear of flying, for example, it may not be possible or even useful to aim at being able to fly to Australia – but you might want to set a realistic goal of flying to your grandson's wedding in *Austria* without having a panic attack.

Time-limited Setting a goal without a realistic time frame can reduce your chances of achieving it. But be careful not to put too much pressure on yourself. 'I want to stop feeling anxious tomorrow' isn't a SMART goal – but 'I want to reduce my anxiety on the Underground journey to work from 9/10 to 4/10 by Christmas' *is* SMART and much more likely to support you in achieving your aim.

You might find these questions helpful in designing your own SMART goal:

- If you achieve what you're hoping for, what will be different?
- How will other people know that you've changed? What will they see you do or hear you say?
- How would you like to think about yourself?

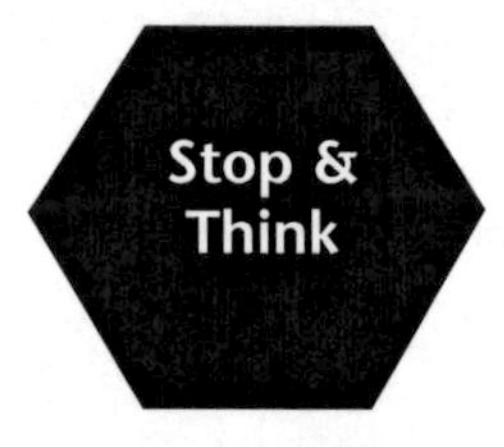

Take time to design your own SMART goal. This could take a while, so you may want a trusted friend or relative to help. When you've written out your goal, decide which technique is most likely to help you. Are you trying to reduce avoidance or safety behaviours, or do you need to use graded exposure? Remember that you may want to start with the techniques in Chapters 7 and 8 first.

This chapter has introduced you to the most important ways of working with what you *do*. We recommend that you glance through the next two chapters before you start to put your first technique into practice – you may find you want to start with learning to relax or working with what you *think*. Whichever technique you start with, use the SMART goal-setting and monitoring to give your hard work the best chance of managing your panic and anxiety.

7

Learning how to relax

Learning relaxation skills is vital for treating panic because it helps you manage the bodily symptoms we've described in this book. These skills will help you gain a sense of control over those unpleasant sensations and enable you to feel more confident. The techniques will also show you that you can cope with difficult situations. Learning how to control physical symptoms of anxiety is a skill that needs to be practised frequently before you can expect lasting benefits and to gain mastery. It's a bit like learning to drive a car. To do that you need to keep practising until you're able to coordinate the many skills required to operate the vehicle without consciously thinking about them. And so with relaxation: it can be a challenge at first, especially if you try to apply the skills in a demanding situation. It's therefore important to start by practising in settings in which you feel comfortable. This chapter will teach you a number of relaxation techniques that will help reduce bodily sensations, stress and tension. We first focus on relaxed, controlled breathing before moving on to teaching you how to release physical tension and relax your body and mind.

Modifying bodily responses

Although the physical experience of fear and panic is normal, it can cause high levels of anxiety if the reaction is misinterpreted or excessive. If your bodily reactions are extreme, the experience can be uncomfortable and distressing enough to give rise to a further challenge that makes the experience of anxiety worse: a fear of experiencing these symptoms. They have the further effect of reinforcing one another. Anticipation of physical discomfort, nausea, sweating, breathing difficulties or tightening in the chest area, to name a few, can then produce the stress that reinforces these bodily sensations. Table 7.1 shows examples of the many exaggerated interpretations of bodily changes.

Table 7.1 Misinterpretations of bodily symptoms

Bodily changes	*What's happening*	*Misinterpretations*
Shallow rapid breathing	Hyperventilation; you're using only the upper parts of the lungs and this results in the inhalation of too much oxygen.	'I can't breathe.' 'I'm suffocating.'
Muscle tightening in the chest area, headaches	Tension; muscular tension causes uncomfortable sensations, such as headaches, tightness in chest area, pains, etc.	'This is a heart attack.' 'I'm having a stroke.'
Nausea and dizziness	When the oxygen level in your body rises (hyperventilation), the relative carbon-dioxide level falls below normal. This imbalance causes unpleasant symptoms, including nausea and light headedness.	'I'll collapse.' 'I'll faint.' 'I'll make a fool of myself.'
Sweating, trembling, hot and flushed	The bodily temperature rises because of physical exertion brought on by hyperventilation and muscular tension.	'I can't cope.' 'I'm weak.'

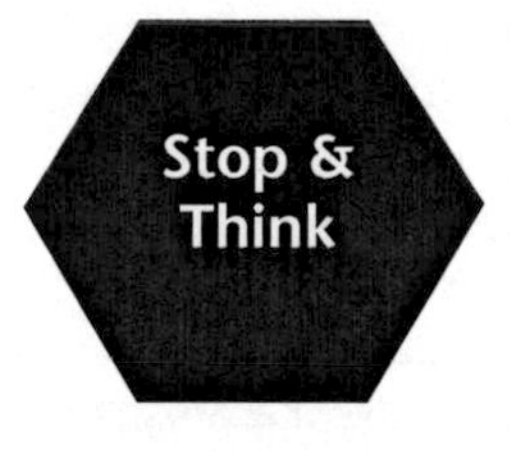

Try to recall the last time you experienced anxiety or panic. Did you notice any changes in your body? If so, what was your immediate interpretation of the physical symptoms? Did your interpretation make you feel better or worse? Was there anything in particular you did to make yourself feel calmer again?

There's a range of techniques that can help you modify the bodily responses associated with panic. We've found relaxed and controlled breathing and applied relaxation to be particularly effective ways of producing physical relief. They're widely recognized methods for coping with bodily sensations during panic attacks, and are designed to tackle hyperventilation (overbreathing) and muscle tension respectively. As we demonstrated in Table 7.1, rapid shallow breathing and muscular tension are thought to maintain and reinforce many of the unpleasant sensations associated with your panic. It therefore makes sense to deal with each of these in turn. You may already be familiar with breathing exercises and healthy ways of resting, especially if you practise yoga or meditation or have completed a course in relaxation skills. If this is the case, the techniques described below can be used to build on existing skills to enhance your repertoire for relaxation.

Relaxed, controlled breathing

We tend to over-breathe whenever we're tense or when we're exercising. This is a mild form of hyperventilation that increases blood circulation so that our muscles can be primed to react during activity. We notice our heart rate increases, our breathing becomes more regular and muscles may tense up slightly. Rapid breathing isn't problematic in the short term – it's a perfectly healthy response to ensure we can sustain exercise, whether working out in the gym, running a marathon or speeding towards the office to make the morning meeting. It's also a normal response to stress and anxiety.

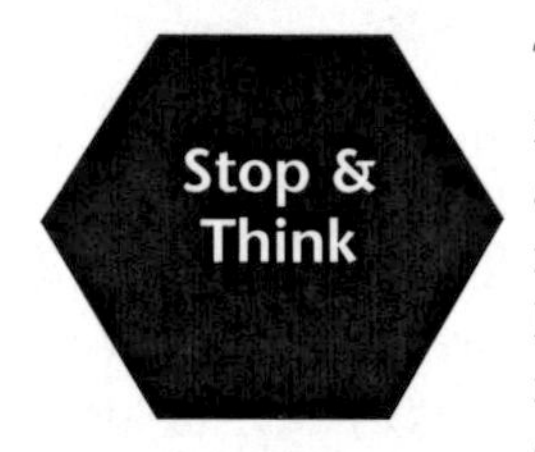

Think about the last time you exercised – a fitness class at your local gym, physical activity with your children in the garden, running to catch a bus perhaps. What happened to your breathing (slower, faster, rapid, shallow)? Did you notice any bodily changes (heavier breathing, increased body temperature, muscle aches especially in the leg area, heart palpitations)? How did you control these physical sensations (slowed down the pace, regular rest periods, deep-breathing techniques)? What happened to your breathing once you stopped exercising or slowed the pace down (continued to over-breathe, found the pace of breathing naturally slowed down)?

Continued rapid breathing can cause intense physical discomfort that can be quite frightening. Imagine that you're sitting at work feeling anxious about leading the morning meeting. Your breathing is getting heavier; you become hot and flushed. You may be thinking, 'What's happening to me?' and 'I'm never going to get through the staff meeting – I'm going to lose control in front of my colleagues.' There are two things happening to your mind and body here: your initial fear of leading the morning meeting has caused over-breathing, which triggers off a range of physical sensations that can be quite uncomfortable. These have led you to develop a second fear: 'I'm going to lose control in front of my colleagues.'

Although it's common to worry that you'll lose control, it's very unlikely you will. It may feel as if the pain will never end, and you may worry that you won't be able to restore healthy breathing. This is a common response to continuous over-breathing. Being able to correct over-breathing is a very powerful way of reducing these unpleasant physical sensations. You can easily learn to do so by developing the habit of 'correct' breathing. Although breathing comes naturally and we all do it without even thinking, there's a tendency to lose our normal ways of breathing when we're afraid, of, for example, having another panic attack, fainting, having a heart attack, losing control or being embarrassed or judged by other people. The breathing technique below will help you develop the ability to control symptoms of over-breathing. You can apply it in almost any situation – during the lead-up to a stressful situation, while feeling anxious or stressed or as a way of controlling physical sensations during a panic attack.

Slowing down your breathing

The overall goal of the breathing technique below is to learn a way to relax through breathing. This involves practising taking gentle, even breaths that fill your lungs completely and exhaling slowly.

You should start by practising in a comfortable setting when you're not too stressed or anxious. Each exercise should last for about ten minutes, and you should ideally practise twice a day – once in the morning, once in the evening. Find a quiet place that's free from distractions and noise. This could be in your office, at home, in the garden or even at your local gym. When you first start practising, you may want to ensure you're alone as it's easy to lose focus – other people may be distracting. You're also more likely to feel self-conscious if your partner or friend is watching when you practise relaxing and controlled breathing for the first time.

- Before you start, it's important you feel comfortable and are able to relax. You can practise controlled breathing in a seated position with your hands relaxed on either side of your body, or in a lying position with your back flat on the ground. If you practise in a lying position, you might find it more comfortable to support your back by placing a pillow or cushion underneath your knees.
- Loosen any tight clothing and take off your shoes if you can.
- Let your shoulder blades sink down your back and lean slightly towards the back of the chair to support your back (or lie flat on your back). Close your eyes.
- Start by taking a deep breath in through your nose and exhale slowly through your mouth. Continue to breathe in through your nose and out through your mouth about five more times.
- Try to make each inhalation and exhalation of the same duration. When you inhale, count slowly from 1 to 4. Do the same when you exhale, so that you're breathing evenly in a slow and focused manner. Notice how your breathing is slowing down.
- Feel the way your lungs gradually expand on every inhalation. As you exhale you're emptying your lungs. Your body feels relaxed. Continue to breathe slowly – in through your nose, out through your mouth.
- Place your right hand on your tummy and let it rest lightly on top of your navel. As you breathe in through your nose, feel the way your tummy rises. As you breathe out through your mouth, your hand is sinking further and further down towards the middle part of your body until your tummy feels completely flat.

- Your heart beat is slowing down. Your arms and legs are relaxed. Continue to count slowly from 1 to 4 on each inhalation and then again for each exhalation.
- On each exhalation, imagine you're pushing the tension out of your lungs. Let it flow through your mouth and out into the wider world. You're getting rid of all the tension, stress and worry.
- Let go of all bodily tension whatsoever. Continue to breathe deeply five more times – in through your nose and out through your mouth. Feel the quietness and peacefulness around you.
- Slowly open your eyes. Continue to breathe gently and evenly, in through your nose and out through your mouth. Softly move your legs and arms. Raise your arms upwards and stretch the whole of your body upwards if you're in a seated position; if you're lying down, flex your arms and legs downwards and gently move back up into a seated position.

Controlled breathing may pose a challenge at first. You may feel as if you're not getting enough air or that the pace of your breathing seems unnaturally slow. This is a normal reaction when you practise a new routine. If you find it difficult to read the instructions while carrying out the breathing routine (most of us do!), you may benefit from recording the instructions with lots of pauses, and playing them back for the first few practices. As your skill improves and you learn to relax quickly, you'll find it easier to switch to correct breathing whenever you feel anxious. You may want to progress to more distracting situations with your eyes open, such as getting the kids off to school! This will improve your skills and help you control your breathing while confronting situations that you fear may increase your panic. The technique is simple and can be used at any stage of a stressful experience to reduce the likelihood of having a panic attack. It's easy to apply and will help reduce tension, anxiety and stress.

Releasing physical tension

Once you've learnt the skill of relaxing your muscles, your mind and body will automatically feel calmer. It's almost impossible for the mind to be tense when the body is relaxed. The ability to relax doesn't always come easily – it's a skill that needs to be learnt gradually and practised regularly. As we've seen, anxiety is different for each of us. We may not have the same bodily symptoms; each of us has our own independent anxious thoughts; each of us behaves differently under stress. It's therefore important that you find a relaxation technique that works for you. This is best done by regular practice before you enter stressful situations that may set off the panic cycle, so that you get used to doing it and gain confidence in its benefits. The aim is to learn relaxation techniques in advance so that you're in a better position to manage bodily sensations during the lead-up to a panic attack. How quickly the physical symptoms of panic can be reduced will vary from person to person. It will depend upon the severity of your panic symptoms, your ability to relax during stress and the nature of muscle tensions involved. Nevertheless, relaxation methods have a very good chance of success if you practise them regularly and take them seriously.

Monitoring progress

Before you begin to practise relaxation skills, spend a minute or two identifying the intensity of your stress and anxiety levels. This

Table 7.2 Measuring your anxiety and stress level

How tense, stressed, and/or anxious do I feel?	*Before relaxation: 1 (low) – 10 (high)*	*After relaxation: 1 (low) – 10 (high)*
Tense		
Stressed		
Anxious		

could be done by asking yourself: 'How tense/stressed/anxious do I feel right now?' Use a scale from 1 (low) to 10 (high) to rate the degree of tenseness/stress/anxiety, as in Table 7.2.

Work through the first of the exercises provided below. Once you've finished, take a further measure of your anxiety. Compare the two sets of scores and see whether you feel less tense/anxious/stressed after completing the relaxation sequence (or no change). Repeat this procedure for each of the exercises provided. You need to know if the relaxation procedure works for you, though there may be some minor variation from day to day.

Progressive muscular relaxation

The first exercise will help you make a distinction between tensed and relaxed muscles. This will help you identify when you're tense so that you can learn to relax your muscles. Muscular tension can occur automatically as a reaction to uncomfortable thoughts and worry. We're not always conscious of physical tension and it's therefore common for people to experience prolonged periods of muscular strain. This exercise will increase your awareness of bodily tension and can therefore act as a cue for when it may be beneficial to apply relaxation techniques to help let go of muscular strain. The sequence is quite simple and takes you through all parts of your body. This exercise is best done in a lying position but if this is difficult, sitting in a chair can work very well. You can use the controlled breathing techniques in the previous exercise to enhance relaxation and calmness. Remember to make a note of how tense/stressed/anxious you are before starting the exercise.

The basic movements you can use for each part of your body are as follows: tense the muscles as much as you can and concentrate on feeling the strain within your body. Hold the tension for about five seconds and then release it. Relax the muscles for 15 seconds and note the difference between their tense and relaxed states. Use this basic technique on each of the muscle groups in turn. Remember to breathe gently and evenly throughout.

Hands Clench your left hand and make a tight fist for 15 seconds. Then relax it for 15 seconds – let it sink towards the ground. Do the same with your right hand.

Arms Tense your whole arm for 15 seconds. Imagine you're holding a set of weights in your hand. Bring the bottom half of your arm upwards as this will make it easier to flex your arm. Relax for 15 seconds. Repeat the process for your right arm.

Face Tense your eyebrows by frowning for 15 seconds, then tense your forehead and jaw. Relax for 15 seconds and repeat.

Neck and shoulders Let your chin drop down towards your chest. Squeeze your shoulders up towards your neck as hard as you can for 15 seconds. Hold for 15 seconds and then relax. Repeat the process one more time. As your shoulders release, feel your shoulder blades slide gently down your back towards your waist.

Abdomen Tighten the muscles in your stomach by pulling them in and up. Hold for 15 seconds and then relax for 15 seconds. Repeat the tensing and relax again.

Thighs Relax your upper body. Tighten your thigh muscles by squeezing your buttocks and thighs together for 15 seconds. Relax for 15 seconds before you repeat the process again.

Legs Bend your feet downwards so that your toes are pointing towards the floor for 15 seconds. There should be a tightening sensation in the back of your leg muscles. Relax for 15 seconds. Then bend your feet the other way so that your toes are pointing upwards. You should feel a light tension in the front part of your legs. Relax.

Whole body Tense all of the above body parts all at once for 15 seconds. You should feel a tension in your hands, face area, neck and shoulders, abdomen, thighs and legs. Relax for 15 seconds and then repeat this process once more.

Take care to not over-tense muscles as this can cause discomfort or even injury. Remember to breathe slowly and regularly between each part of the exercise. When you've finished the sequence, spend a minute or two thinking about something pleasant. For example, a relaxing walk along the seafront or eating a piece of your favourite chocolate cake. This can allow for a gentle transition back into your normal environment again. Before you stand up straight, gently stretch and move your arms and legs and avoid sudden or jerky movements. When you're ready, take your time standing up. If you still feel tense at the end of the exercise, try to go through the sequence once more. Remember: it takes time to learn how to relax. Give yourself a chance and don't expect to succeed too soon.

Once you've mastered the muscle-relaxing exercise above, you can shorten it by missing out the tensing stage. You can go through the routine systematically by focusing on each of the muscle groups for 15–20 seconds at a time. You can adapt the exercise so that you can do it while at work, at home, during train journeys or just about anywhere else. If you're used to practising relaxation skills in a 'heavenly calm sanctuary', you may be put off by the external distractions of everyday living, such as traffic noise, sounds of people chatting/phones ringing in your office or children crying at home. Learning to relax in a range of different environments is important because this is what you need for coping in the real world. You can use relaxation skills whenever you feel anxious, stressed or panicky.

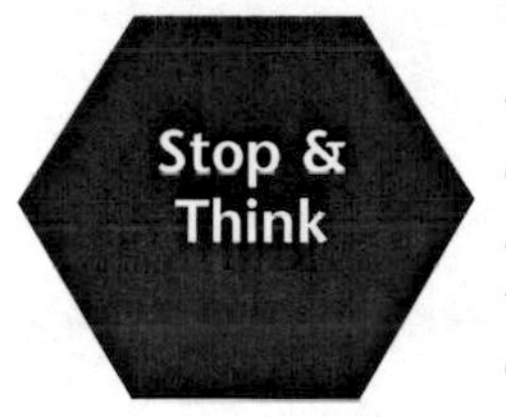

Remember to monitor your progress. Use the before-and-after table (Table 7.2) to ensure that you compare your level of anxiety before and after you've completed the exercise. This will also help you find out which type of relaxation works best for you.

Deep relaxation

For this exercise, you'll need to imagine a soothing, restful situation to use during the sequence. The mental image will help you relax even more effectively. This exercise is a form of distraction and can help you learn to calm yourself down. You may need to practise the sequence a number of times. This will help you use a mental image to relax yourself whenever you feel stressed or anxious. Before you start the exercise, remember to note your anxiety/tension level and compare at the end. Here are some suggestions for mental images to help you get started.

- A particular place you've visited that you associate with peacefulness and calmness. A deserted beach, your holiday home, your garden, the views from the top of a mountain, watching the rain run down your window, the scenery during a visit to the countryside.
- A poem, lyric of a song, a word or a catchphrase that brings positive images to your mind.
- A pleasant object, person, film or picture you particularly like.

When you've decided what mental image you'll use, follow the instructions below. Again, it may be useful to record these, including lots of pauses, and to play the recording back to guide your first few practice sessions.

- Sit in a comfortable position with your eyes closed.
- Start by focusing on your breathing – listen to the sounds of your breaths.
- When you inhale, fill the lungs completely before you exhale by slowly letting go of the air. Slow the breathing down.
- As you continue to breathe, focus on your mental image; the things that you can see, hear and smell. Simply let go of all tension and allow your mind and body to relax.
- Feel your body growing heavier and heavier. Stay with the image and continue to breathe naturally and steadily. Keep the exercise going for 15–20 minutes.

When you've finished, open your eyes and sit in the same position for a minute or two. Slowly move your limbs and prepare yourself to stand up.

Regular exercise

Another way to become more relaxed is to engage in regular exercise. Exercise helps your body relieve tension caused by anxiety and stress. There are many forms of exercise of course, some lighter than others. They could include going for a brisk walk, walking up a set of stairs as opposed to taking the lift/escalator, going to the gym, going for a run, mountain walking, cycling, ballroom dancing and attending a yoga class – to name but a few.

The positive effects of regular exercise

- Regular exercise can have a positive effect on your mood – it stimulates various brain chemicals, which can leave you feeling happier and more relaxed than you were before you worked out.
- Regular exercise delivers blood, oxygen and nutrients to your tissues – in fact it helps your entire cardiovascular system work more efficiently.
- Regular exercise can help you fall asleep faster and deepen your sleep.
- Regular exercise has a positive effect on your health, weight and overall vitality.

You can start exercising by setting yourself small goals, such as walking to the shops instead of driving, signing up for gym classes at your local leisure centre or digging your bicycle out of the garage and checking if it still works.

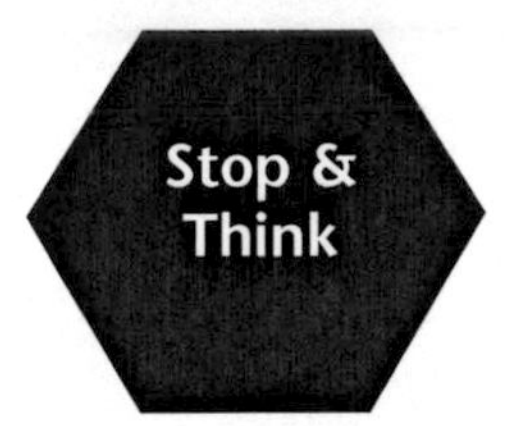

What type of physical exercise do you want to/could you do (walking, jogging, cycling, dancing, climbing)? Think about a time of the day and week that would be most convenient to start exercising. What may be stopping you from doing physical exercise (health concerns, lack of time, lack of motivation, fear of looking or feeling stupid, needing to buy sport equipment)? Try to think about ways to overcome these obstacles and implement your solutions accordingly (getting health clearance from your GP, join a dance class with a friend to increase your motivation).

Learning how to relax is a skill that can help reduce the bodily symptoms of panic. As we've said, you may need to practise controlled breathing and relaxation several times before you will fully discover their effectiveness. They're an important part of managing your bodily symptoms and so can help reduce physical distress and the uncomfortable sensations of panic.

8

Managing fears and worries about having a panic attack

Worrying thoughts about what might happen to you are a major contribution to panic. In the first section of this chapter, we list a number of common worries likely to make us think in a way that often makes our panic worse. The aim is to encourage you to begin to examine your own thinking so that you can start the process of managing your fears. This theme will be explored further in Chapter 9, which teaches you a number of practical techniques for challenging and changing worrying thoughts. Another key aspect of overcoming your panic is to learn how to focus less on bodily sensations, so that you can build a more balanced, and perhaps more accurate, picture of the state of your body and physical wellbeing. Learning to focus your attention on what's happening outside of yourself, instead of what's happening inside, will help you become less focused on your body and feel more confident and secure about common bodily sensations. The second part of this chapter will teach you how to do this.

Learning to examine your thoughts

We now turn to your own thoughts about panic. A very common factor in panic is the way people sometimes think about the physical sensations produced by anxiety or changes in them by things like running for a bus or doing an exercise class. Changes in heart rate, breathing, palpitations or even muscle tension can make people who are particularly sensitive to these changes think that something dreadful is happening to them. This way of thinking, which we call catastrophizing, will almost certainly make you feel anxious and is often a driving force in panic. To manage this, the first step is learning to recognize what you're thinking.

Let's start by identifying your thoughts about the particular fears that may be underlying your panic attacks. Discovering your key thoughts can be more difficult than you think. They are more often than not automatic thoughts that reside in our mind – you may not be conscious of them because you're either so used to, or very good at, suppressing them. A good way to identify underlying fears is to pay attention to emotional changes and use these as a cue for paying attention to your thinking. If you notice any anxiety or tension when you think about a panic-inducing situation, such as going on public transport, sitting an exam or going to a concert, stop whatever you're doing (if possible) and ask yourself: 'What am I thinking about right now?' To start with, identify three or four thoughts that worry you most about the particular situation, place or person in question, and make a note of them. You could use Table 8.1 to structure your worry.

Table 8.1 Identifying your worry

Situation	*Feeling*	*Worrying thought*
Working late in the office – noticing discomfort/pain in the heart area	Anxious	'I'm having a heart attack.'
Going to a concert – standing in the middle of a crowd and starting to hyperventilate	Scared	'I'm suffocating.'
Add your own here		

The following are some common examples of thoughts that make people afraid.

'I'm going to have a panic attack and faint in public.'

Obviously people do sometimes faint, but it is rare and mostly happens because their blood pressure drops, reducing the blood supply to the brain. There are other reasons why people faint, some of which may be linked to medical illness, temperature or oxygen levels. The worst thing that usually happens is that a person may fall over, but they quickly come around and gain consciousness, unless of course they're injured when they collapse. When you panic, the heart pumps harder and faster than usual and the blood pressure actually rises. This is the opposite of a faint, which is why it's almost impossible to faint when you're panicking! However, people who have a specific fear of blood or injections, called blood-injury phobia, react differently in that their blood pressure drops when they're confronted with one of their fears.

'I won't be able to sit in a small, closed room on this train, or be in a crowded place, because I won't get enough air – I'll suffocate!'

It's true that crowded, hot or small places or rooms without ventilation can feel less comfortable, but this doesn't mean you'll get less air. When we breathe in, our bodies only use a small amount of oxygen, and even in a small room there's a large amount of air The other point worth remembering is that most of the rooms we use in everyday life aren't as airtight as we might think – air is invisible and flows in and out at a much faster speed than we can use it up. There's therefore no risk of suffocation even if you feel uncomfortable.

'I've lost all control – I'm going mad!'

Although it may feel as if you're 'going mad', it's worth learning more about mental illness. Broadly speaking, there are two different kinds of psychological disorders. The first type, neurotic problems, are common disorders that can happen to everyone, and include anxiety and panic, post-traumatic stress and most depressive disorders, to name a few. The second type, psychoses, are less common and include such severe mental illnesses as psychotic episodes and schizophrenia. People with panic are no more likely than anyone else to develop severe mental illnesses, and most neurotic disorders are treatable using self-help, psychological therapy or medication. Panic is often associated with a fear of loss of control, which isn't really indicative of severe mental illness.

'I feel tense and nervous – I'm going to have a panic attack.'

You think something catastrophic will happen, such as having a panic attack, because you feel tense and nervous. You act upon your feelings or physical symptoms and let these control your understanding of the environment. Most often we tend to fear that some disaster is more likely to happen, and be much worse, than it actually is. For example, you may think that you'll have a panic attack while travelling on the train, and that you'll lose control and try to jump out of the train while it's in fast motion. You may ignore the fact that you might not have a panic attack at all, that if you were to you'd be able to control yourself just as you've done every time you felt panicky, or that the panicky feeling will eventually pass. Unfortunately, thinking errors such as catastrophizing are likely to exacerbate avoidance and unhelpful behaviours because they prevent people from daring to confront panic-inducing situations.

Redirecting your attention

Now that we've emphasized how what you think can contribute to feelings of panic, we'll introduce you to one way of managing these thoughts: learning to pay less attention to them and distracting yourself.

Distraction or attentional training often works well as a way of coping with an anxious situation. When we consciously look for bodily changes or we're highly 'tuned in' to them, we're likely to become more aware of bodily sensations that we may not otherwise have noticed. This could trigger further worry and anxiety, which in turn could amplify physical sensations. Worrying about anxiety and fearing panic attacks are common triggers of panic, even if it's not what we want to happen. This section will teach you to direct your attention away from your bodily symptoms and to reduce self-monitoring, and instead to focus on the external environment. Learning to control your attention is an effective way to reduce sensitivity to bodily sensations.

We all experience bodily changes on a daily basis, but because they're so common we usually don't notice them – for example, changes to our body temperature, the rhythm of our breathing and the pace of our heart beats. But if you consciously start to look out for them, you may suddenly become aware of symptoms you otherwise wouldn't have noticed. Let's take an unrelated example: you may have had the experience of wanting to go to a particular destination for a holiday. Suddenly you see adverts of your dream holiday destination in several different places – on the television, in magazines and on billboards. It's likely that the adverts were there before, but because you didn't place importance on going on holiday until recently, you may not have consciously noticed them.

We tend to notice only things that are important to us. It's the same with bodily sensations. They're always there but ordinarily we don't pay much attention to them. The problem with too much focus on bodily sensations is that once you start looking for changes, you may pay so much attention to what are perfectly normal ones that you become anxious or panicky. This could increase your worry and stress, which could make you more susceptible to a panic attack. This is what happened in the case below, where you'll see that Jennifer's catastrophic interpretation of bodily sensations and the way she reacted to physical symptoms of stress contributed towards panic.

Jennifer, a 45-year-old barrister, had a panic attack in her office while working late one evening preparing for a difficult court case (**situation**). It began with an unusual 'butterfly' sensation in the chest area. She felt increasingly hot, especially in her legs and feet (**physical sensations**). She thought she was going to faint. Her heart was racing and she was convinced there was something seriously wrong with her health (**misinterpretations of bodily sensations**). She asked her clerk to call a taxi, which took her to the nearest hospital (**action taken based on misinterpretation**). After examination, the doctor told Jennifer that there were no indications of physical illness. He thought she'd suffered a panic attack and explained the link between anxiety and physical sensations. Work stress was the likely cause. Jennifer recalled feeling frightened that she'd experience another panic attack at work (**fear of having another panic attack in the future**). She started to scan her body on a daily basis to ensure there were 'no signs of unusual sensations in the heart area' (**overly sensitive to bodily changes**). Sometimes she'd find a slight irregularity in her heart beat (**normal changes**). This would often cause her to worry about having another panic attack. Consequently she'd often sit down on the floor to avoid fainting or falling over in case her legs gave way (**safety behaviours**). She also stopped taking on difficult cases, fearing doing so might set off another panic attack (**avoidance**).

Worry is a natural state in anticipation of risk, and it keeps us safe from danger and catastrophe. When our perception of risk is raised or exaggerated, we're also likely to feel unsafe and hence start to worry to protect ourselves from the imagined fear. This is why anxious thoughts about bodily sensations can be intense and persistent. The challenge here is to let go of your worry because it makes you focus too much on your body and also interferes with your ability to act, think and feel in a rational way.

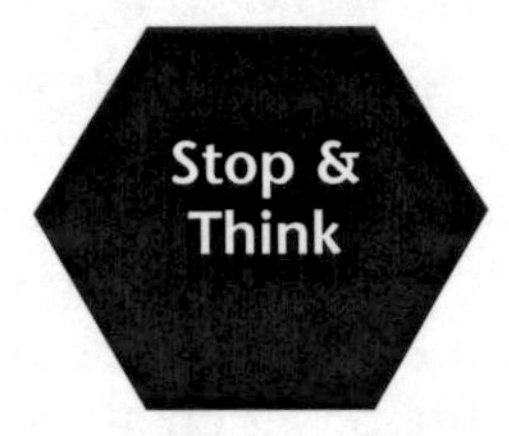

Anxious thoughts can make you feel distressed and overwhelmed. They're often characterized by uncertainty and tend to beg a number of 'What if . . .?' questions. Some people say anxious thoughts are like a 'stuck record': it feels like the same words are being repeated over and over again in their minds. This is an ideal time to practise distraction techniques. By concentrating on something else, you can stop paying attention to your anxious thoughts, which will allow you to feel more comfortable and relaxed. Try to identify the distractions most likely to work for you. Read through the rest of this chapter and pick the technique that most appeals to you or seems most likely to be effective. Do work through the instructions for that technique in detail and try it for yourself. If after a reasonable amount of practice it's not working as well as you'd like, try another one. Plan to use your individual distraction technique next time you feel anxious.

The concentration techniques we'll describe will help you stop the flow of anxious thoughts, reduce your distress and make you feel more calm and relaxed. They'll also help you direct your attention away from your body so that you can focus on the external environment. You may want to start practising while you're feeling calm and relaxed. Once you develop your ability to direct your attention away from your body, you can move on to use the techniques during more challenging situations.

Listening to the lyrics of a song

Select a song you like and play it. Concentrate on the lyrics for about two minutes. Turn off the song and summarize the lyrics of the song out loud. Note how much of your attention is directed towards the task of listening to the song, yourself and the environment around you. You can use percentage to measure the focus of your attention. The result might come out something like Table 8.2.

Table 8.2 Attentional training (1)

Concentrating on task	*Concentrating on yourself*	*Concentrating on environment*
40%	30%	30%

Carry out the exercise again but choose a different song. Deliberately try to distract yourself this time by focusing on your thoughts and sensations before you redirect your concentration towards the lyrics of the song. Summarize the lyrics again and note how you divided your attention between your thoughts, sensations and the task of listening to the song. Use Table 8.3 to add your own data in percentage, as shown previously.

Table 8.3 Attentional training (2)

Concentrating on task	*Concentrating on your thoughts*	*Concentrating on your sensations*

Repeat the listening activities until you become adept at redirecting your attention to the task of listening to the words of the song after deliberate distraction through focusing on yourself. This will help develop your ability to control where and when you focus your attention.

Paying attention to your immediate surroundings

This exercise asks you to pay attention to the entireness of your surroundings – what you can see, feel, hear and smell. The value of this is to help you shift your focus away from bodily sensations towards the more pleasant and positive aspects of your surroundings. You can use almost any situation to practise shifting your attention towards the outside world. This includes walking to your local food store, a trip in the park, attending a social event, visiting a museum, travelling to work or making a special meal.

- Focus your attention for about six minutes on the different aspects of your surroundings.
- Now, focus your attention on mainly what you can see – colours, objects and people.
- After about one minute, begin to shift your attention towards what you can hear – the various noises around you.
- Then shift your attention to concentrate on smells, before you redirect the focus towards your feelings.
- Keep moving your attention around to these different sensations. Try to vary the order of your attention to the individual sensations as this will help develop your skills for controlling your attention. Notice how you feel much more relaxed once you direct your attention away from yourself.
- Next, try to integrate your attention to include all aspects of your surroundings. Notice how much you're paying attention to the different aspects of the environment – what you can see, feel, hear and smell.

Choosing where to focus your attention

Another way to reduce the extent to which you may be focused on your internal thoughts, emotions and physical sensations is to practise using the majority of your attention in a way you choose. With practice, being able to do this in situations where you may become anxious means you can reduce the impact the unpleasant sensations of panic have on you. This does take quite a lot of practice to master but is often well worth the effort. You'll then be able to choose to direct your attention to the more pleasant aspects of anxiety-provoking situations – what people are talking about, the taste of good food and so on.

- Start by finding a time and place where you can try this technique for a short period. You need several sounds to practise focusing on, so may want to use a room where there's some external noise, such as traffic or people walking outside, and some internal, perhaps a clock ticking and an electric fan.
- Choose a noise in the room and do your best to focus on it for 20 seconds – you should find you notice very little of the other internal noises or any external noise while you do this.
- Focus on another noise in the room for 20 seconds – you probably won't hear the first noise you focused on while doing this. Try to focus on an external noise for 20 seconds – you should find you barely notice the internal sounds.
- Don't spend too long practising this skill to start with – paying attention for 20 seconds to each of three of four different sounds and then repeating that once is enough. When you can confidently do that, extend the time you focus on each to 40 seconds and then to a minute.

When you're confident you can choose where to focus your attention on your own, try the same exercise when you're with other people. When approaching a stressful situation, you can use those techniques to help prevent yourself from engaging with the anxious thoughts that often trigger panic. Focusing too much on bodily changes makes you increasingly aware of physical sensations, feelings, thoughts and behaviours. This can lead to negative interpretations of normal changes in your body, which in turn may trigger panic and anxiety. By consciously focusing on people and external aspects outside of yourself, you'll feel less distressed and allow yourself to be in touch with what's happening around you. With practice you can train yourself to tune into the external world even when you're feeling anxious.

Other distraction techniques

There are a number of additional techniques that can help you take your mind off physical sensations of panic. You may already have found distraction techniques that work for you, and we encourage you to continue using them in addition to attention redirection. Below is a list of suggestions for other ways to help you distract yourself from bodily sensations and anxiety-provoking thoughts.

- Listen to your favourite band, classical music, songs and so on.
- Go for a walk, run or engage in some other light exercise. Research shows that exercise helps release natural endorphins, a chemical in the brain area known to have a positive impact on mood. When we feel positive we're less likely to think negatively and therefore less prone to misinterpretations of bodily symptoms. Exercise can also buffer against stress and is especially effective for relieving muscular tension.
- Read a book or magazine you find interesting – you're more likely to sustain attention on topics that appeal to you.
- Enrol on a course of yoga or meditation. You may find it difficult to focus all your attention on the sessions at first but this is completely normal when you're learning a new skill. Many people say they've found yoga and meditation helpful for dealing with stress, anxiety and panic.
- Arrange a visit to a place you'd like to explore, such as somewhere in the UK countryside, a town, the museum, theatre or any other venues of interest. If you don't feel like travelling, finding a calming place in your house could work equally well – the most important thing is to feel relaxed.
- Talk to a friend, partner or family member – this may help take your mind off your panic. Although it can be helpful to discuss your panic symptoms with a friend, take care not to bring them up too much in case you adversely reinforce your panic, first by drawing attention to your symptoms and second, by falling into the trap of seeking reassurance from others. You may wish to restrict most conversations to topics independent of your panic. Talking with others about your anxiety or panic can have different effects – a measure of calm because you feel understood and connected to another person, or an increase in anxiety because you're giving the problem more attention and focus. It's not always possible to predict the specific effect or outcome.

9

How can thinking help me manage a panic attack?

Almost everyone who wants to manage their panic needs to learn to relax and work on what they do and what they think. This chapter describes more skills and techniques for working with what you think. The skills presented here are about challenging unhelpful ways of thinking. We especially focus on how you might think about physical symptoms of anxiety, which are often a major contributing factor to panic.

Can I really change what I think?

It may seem daunting or even impossible to change the way you think. First, remember that what we're asking you to do is learn a new skill. Think back to learning to ride a bicycle, drive a car or starting a new hobby. Most people need a lot of practice to become skilled at anything. Managing the way you think involves learning another new skill, and nobody will be perfect at it to start with. Second, you'll find as you work through this chapter that the techniques are about spotting and challenging unhelpful ways of thinking. The aim isn't to control what you think; rather it's to identify and then alter unhelpful ways of thinking when they do happen so that you can change how you feel and manage your panic more effectively.

The basic steps in managing thoughts that may drive anxiety and panic are:

1. noticing thoughts that make you feel anxious;
2. checking how accurate those thoughts are;
3. if they're accurate, using techniques that may help to focus on what you do, especially learning to counter the physical sensations of panic with relaxation techniques;

4 if your thinking isn't completely accurate, using the techniques in this chapter to challenge them and monitor the effect that has on your anxiety.

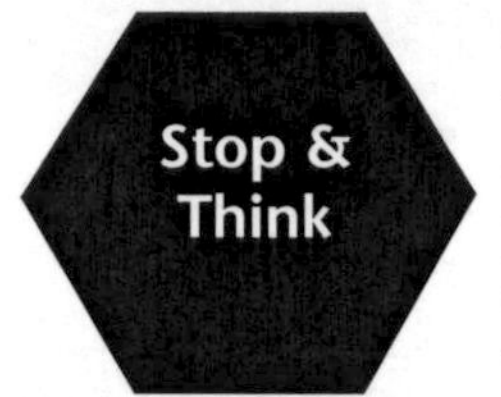

Chapter 8 asked you to notice the thoughts that may contribute to your anxiety. Take a few minutes now to go back to the notes you made as you worked through that chapter. What are the most important thoughts to work with first?

Noticing thoughts that make you feel anxious

Working through the earlier parts of this book you'll have gained a good understanding of the ways you tend to think that may be a significant part of what drives your panic. The starting point is to notice these thoughts and the context in which they occur, such as the places, people or events that trigger them. It's also important to identify the way these thoughts make you feel. If you're finding it difficult to identify them, you might find it helpful to remember a time when you were feeling panic or extremely anxious and ask yourself these questions:

- When did I first notice that I felt anxious? Where was I, what was I doing and who was there?
- What was going through my mind (it may have been thoughts, pictures or moving images or just a sense of dread)?
- What was it about when, where, what and who at that time and place that made me think that?
- What did that thought or image make me feel?
- If you can only remember the feeling of panic at first, you might ask yourself what happened to trigger that feeling. What made you anxious about that?

If you find it difficult to identify the thoughts that you want to work with, you might like to carry a notebook with you for a few days and record situations that make you anxious. Remember that sometimes our thoughts relate to what we think might happen ('I'm going to have a heart attack'). At others they relate to what we think is happening ('I'm going mad').

Checking how accurate your thoughts are

When we concentrate on trying to get something right or appearing skilled and confident, we tend not to pay much attention to what we're thinking. That means that the thoughts that initially drive anxiety and even panic may go unnoticed. When trying to treat panic, it's important to notice these thoughts and check how accurate they are. Many people find it much easier to identify the evidence that supports unhelpful thoughts than evidence that might contradict that way of thinking. These questions might help you identify evidence that doesn't support thoughts that make you feel anxious:

- Can you think of any experiences that show that thought isn't completely correct at all times?
- If a good friend or loved one thought this way, what would you say to them?
- What did other people actually say about the situation that caused you to panic?

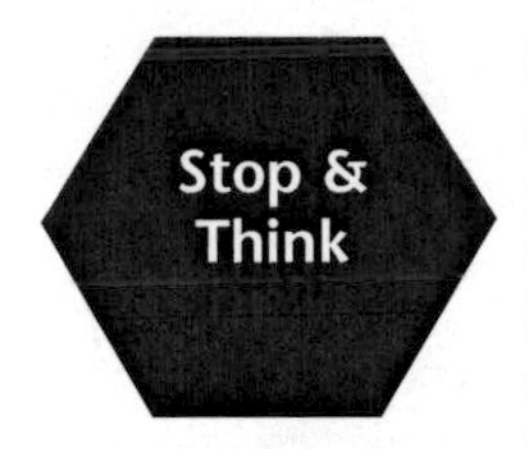

Do you notice how almost all these sources of evidence are based on what other people think? Often people who've learnt to become anxious or to panic have become very good at thinking in a particular way that drives their anxiety. Take a few moments to think about who you could ask for objective feedback on situations where you feel anxious, or what evidence you could gather about the unhelpful thoughts you've amassed so far.

Working with the evidence for and against unhelpful thoughts

It's important not to rush gathering evidence to support or challenge the way you think. Once you've collected all the evidence you can, look through it as objectively as possible. It may help if you ask someone you trust to do this with you to start with. If you do, explain that you need them to be objective. They'll want to support you and may worry about hurting your feelings if they can identify evidence that backs up your upsetting thoughts. (They may find it helpful to look through Chapter 10 first.) We often find it's particularly beneficial to remind someone who wants to help that you need to understand how accurate your thoughts are so you can decide how to work with them. If your thoughts are accurate and upsetting, it simply means you need to work with what you *do* rather than what you *think*.

As you look at the evidence you've collected about a thought, ask yourself the following questions:

- Is there more evidence for or more against that way of thinking?
- When I look at the evidence objectively, how accurate is that thought?
- Is there another way to think about it?

Once you've taken the time to look at the evidence in detail, you'll often see that the thought that makes you feel anxious or even panic isn't completely accurate.

Constructing alternative ways of thinking

The final step in working with unhelpful thoughts is to practise alternative ways of thinking about the situations that triggered them. Again, this takes practice and can seem challenging at first – you may want to ask someone you trust to help. The most important thing to remember is that we're not asking you to come up with 'empty' positive ways of thinking. Any alternative must be based on the evidence you collected when challenging this thought – it has to be realistic. Then notice how the alternative way of thinking makes you feel.

We introduced some common thoughts that often contribute to panic in Chapter 8. Table 9.1 shows some alternative ways of thinking that many people have found useful in overcoming panic.

When trying to construct alternative ways of thinking in difficult situations, start by taking an objective look at all the evidence you've gathered. Does it really prove that the thoughts you're working with are completely true all the time? The following questions and list of examples may also help:

- What would somebody who was confident in that situation be thinking?
- Remember that panic is often driven by thoughts about physical sensations in your body. Are you reacting in this way to physical sensations that are the result of anxiety or exercise (if this is the case, you'll almost certainly need to learn to relax to control those physical reactions as well as work with what you think)?
- Was I so focused on the fact that I felt anxious, awkward or

Table 9.1 Common thoughts that drive panic, and alternative ways of thinking

Thought	*Evidence against*	*Alternative thought*
'I'm going to have a panic attack and faint in public.'	Remember that a panic attack causes high blood pressure, which means you won't faint.	'This might be uncomfortable but I can manage that with controlled breathing and relaxation, and I'm unlikely to faint.'
'I won't be able to sit in a small, closed room on this train, or be in a crowded place because I won't get enough air – I'll suffocate!'	There's enough air for everyone even in a crowded train, although it may not be pleasant.	'The train is hot and uncomfortable but I can breathe and it's only a short journey. I'm looking forward to getting home.'
'I've lost all control – I'm going mad!'	Panic is frightening and unpleasant but it doesn't mean you're going mad.	'This is panic and I'm beginning to learn how to manage it. It won't last long.'
'I feel tense and nervous – I'm going to have a panic attack.'	You probably haven't panicked every time you felt this way.	'Even if I do panic, I've learned ways of managing that, and it won't last long.'
'I'm having a heart attack!'	What might have caused your heart rate to increase? Have you been exercising or has something made you anxious?	'My heart is racing because I just ran for the bus. I've checked with my doctor and these symptoms are normal.'

stupid that I didn't notice that at least some people reacted positively to me or what I was saying?
- If I received formal or informal feedback from other people, what did they think was good about what I did?
- Even if I feel nervous, awkward or physically sick, does it really last forever?
- When I look back in five years' time, how important will that situation be?

Using alternative ways of thinking

When you've spotted a thought related to your anxiety that's inaccurate and unhelpful, and have designed an alternative thought, the final step in breaking the vicious cycle of anxiety is to practise using that thought. Having worked through this book, you'll realize this means you'll need to practise your new way of thinking actively. There are several ways you might do this:

- Write or print your new thought on a card that you keep with you. Read it to yourself or even out loud when you notice yourself becoming anxious.
- In a similar way, you could use 'cue cards' like this at home, in the office or even in the car (not to be read while driving though!). If you don't want everyone to see them, you could keep copies in the tops of drawers or inside cupboard doors.
- Share your new way of thinking with a trusted friend or relative and ask them to remind you to use it if they see you becoming anxious.

Putting it all together

Overcoming panic and anxiety means that you need to break your unique vicious cycle of panic. Many people select which technique they work with first by identifying the point at which they'd like to break into their anxious cycle. For example, if you notice that you start to worry that you might be about to panic when you have a particular thought, you might want to break into that cycle by working with an alternative thought. The aim in doing that would be to change the emotions associated with whatever triggered that thought, which in turn should have an impact on what you do (perhaps starting to do something you'd been avoiding) and your physical reactions to that trigger. In this case, changing what you think has had an impact on how you feel (physically and emotionally) and what you do.

It's also possible to learn to manage panic by using what you do to influence what you think and how you feel. We demonstrated how this might work when we described using graded exposure (Chapter 6) or reducing the extent to which you avoid whatever triggers your anxiety (Chapter 5). Effectively, you're challenging thoughts such as, 'I'll panic' or, 'This is frightening' by doing something that demonstrates that the thought isn't completely accurate. Similarly, learning to relax can challenge the thought, 'I can't control my panic'. Both these ways of working should then have an impact on how you feel.

Essentially, all this means is that once you can map out your unique cycle of panic, you can start breaking into it at any stage. If the technique you try first isn't effective at managing all four aspects of panic (thoughts, behaviours, physical sensations and emotions), you may need to add another technique to reinforce its effect or break into another part of your panic cycle. Here are two final vignettes to illustrate what we mean:

> Clare had learnt to think, 'I'm certain to panic' when she had to travel by Underground. This thought would make her feel anxious and her body would react by trembling. She'd start to hyperventilate and would, indeed, often panic. When she talked to a friend who'd previously struggled with panic, he pointed out that she could sometimes make the journey to work without panicking. He suggested she have a cue card in her pocket with the alternative thought: 'I can cope with the journey to work'. Clare thought this was fantastic and it worked for four days in a row – she'd read it to herself just as she entered the station at the start of her journey. Unfortunately, on Friday morning the Underground was particularly crowded. Clare began to feel hot and her breathing started to become shallow and rapid. She quickly found herself in a full-blown panic attack and went home, from where she rang work to say she was ill.
>
> Eventually Clare's GP referred her to a psychologist. Together they worked out that although Clare's alternative thought did have a positive effect on her anxiety, it didn't have an impact on the way she reacted

to physical sensations related to anxiety. Clare learned relaxation and breathing techniques to control these symptoms and created a new alternative thought: 'If I start to feel anxious I can use what I've learnt to manage how I feel'. This combination proved very effective at overcoming her panic.

Clare learned that being able to do something to manage her physical symptoms backed up and increased the effect of a new way of thinking.

Mark would think, 'I'm going to fall and die' when he was at any height – buildings, ladders and tall hills all posed a significant challenge. Working with a counsellor, he used graded exposure to improve his confidence. He'd still shake when climbing ladders though. He needed a lot of practice at learning to relax his physical tension. This eventually changed what he'd think to: 'I'm getting good at managing my tendency to shake and I'll be safe for the short time I'm at this height'. Once he'd achieved this, Mark became much more confident at being in high places or using ladders, and was able to take his children to the top of the local church tower and enjoy the view from there.

Mark used a combination of doing something and learning to relax to manage his panic. In doing this he discovered that what he thought changed as well.

Realistic alternative ways of thinking can have a significant impact on our emotions and the way our bodies respond to experiences that trigger panic. It often takes practice both to construct the alternative thoughts and to use them in challenging situations. Remember that you may have had years of practice in unhelpful ways of thinking, and it will take time to recognize and change those thoughts.

Summary

There's a lot of information in this chapter and you may need to come back to it more than once. Essentially, we've shown you there are ways you can change how you feel by working with what you think. The basic steps are:

1 Identify the situations you find difficult and make a note of what you think then and how that makes you feel.

2 Take an objective look at those thoughts. Can you see any thinking errors? What's the evidence?
3 If the thinking isn't completely accurate, how else could you think about the evidence you've collected? Practise that new way of thinking and notice how it makes you feel.
4 When you've constructed an alternative thought, it takes practice to use it effectively. Often it works best in combination with managing what you do.

10

How to help a friend or relative with panic attacks

Many clients we treat for panic attacks describe how difficult it can be for others to understand how to help them. If a close friend or family member suffers from panic attacks there are several challenges that he or she may face. Having a supportive family and network of friends can make it easier to cope with and overcome extreme anxiety. For a start, gaining support and feeling understood can help reduce your fears, embarrassment and sense of shame. Having a panic attack may make close family and friends feel more anxious: they may feel they may be 'contaminated' or become 'infected' with the same anxiety you experience. While it's impossible for real contamination to happen, it's easy to see how some of the extreme and unpleasant symptoms associated with panic attacks can leave people around you feeling stressed, worried and uncertain how best to help.

It's not always easy for family members or friends to know exactly what they should do. They may be uncertain whether to react as though it were a medical emergency and to call for immediate assistance. They may fear something unpleasant and life-threatening is happening to you, and feel unskilled or ill-prepared to help you. Alternatively, for others it may be 'just' another episode or instance of your having a panic attack, and they may feel more confident in knowing how to provide immediate support. The first thing they can do to help is take your symptoms seriously and at all costs avoid telling you to 'Snap out of it' or 'Stop breathing so erratically' and so on. However, they'll be unhelpful if they're completely overcome with anxiety themselves or fully collude with your tendency to shun away from situations you find particularly stressful. This chapter will show friends and relatives how to support someone who becomes anxious or panicky, using the techniques described in this book. If you've worked through it and want to ask a friend or relative to help you put the techniques into practice, you could start by lending this book to them and suggesting he or she read this chapter first. If you're trying to support someone who's asked you for help in reducing his or her panic attacks, or in coping better with them, this chapter is a good starting point.

If a friend or relative has asked you to help with a problem such as their coping with panic attacks, you may feel overwhelmed or think you've no idea what to do. Perhaps it's a problem you've experienced yourself at some point and haven't been able to overcome. You may feel helpless when your friend or relative panics and worry you won't be able to help. This chapter is written for you, to give some precise ways of providing support – but there's a lot of information in the rest of the book that may also be useful in helping to understand your friend's or relative's difficulties. He or she could suggest which chapters would be most useful and teach you about his or her unique experience of anxiety and panic attacks.

If you do feel overwhelmed, remember that panic attacks are a treatable psychological condition – unless you're a qualified therapist or psychologist it would be unreasonable to expect you to deliver 'therapy'!

You may need to encourage your friend or relative to seek professional help, and after this chapter we provide a list of relevant organizations that could help you establish a link with a suitable therapist. Remember, however, that panic attacks are often unpredictable and may occur seemingly spontaneously. At the time of their occurrence the person affected may not feel able, confident or resourceful enough to talk about the experience, let alone think about contacting a professional for help. Your friend's or relative's levels of distress may prevent him or her from taking the necessary steps to reduce the symptoms and seek to overcome the problem. He or she may also feel embarrassed or ashamed of having a panic attack and the apparent loss of self-control. However, as a close friend or relative, the fact that you're aware of the problem – either because you've witnessed it or talked about it together – suggests you may have a positive role to play in helping. This is a good starting point.

A brief introduction to panic attacks

There are a variety of ways to support somebody who experiences panic attacks. The most effective way will of course depend on the particular situation that triggers the panic attack. No two people are exactly the same, and it's therefore important to understand that not everyone who suffers from panic attacks describes the same cause or trigger or the same underlying difficulties. Laura's experience is but one example of how panic attacks occur:

> Laura was at a parents' evening for her youngest son when she suddenly began to feel hot and clammy. She noticed tightness in the chest area and it was becoming increasingly difficult to breathe. It felt as if the small office belonging to her son's form tutor were closing in on her. She tried to listen to Mr Lee's academic evaluation of her son but kept missing some of the words because she was so worried about her breathing. She kept thinking to herself that she'd be OK as soon as she could get some fresh air outside the room. She tried to slow down her breathing, hoping this might help her calm down. Mr Lee was getting up to fetch the rest of her son's school report when he became aware of Laura's distressed state. He was surprised at how pale her face had become and asked her if she was all right. Laura wanted to put a brave face on it and opened her mouth to say she was perfectly fine, when she noticed that her whole body had started shaking. In a calm manner, Mr Lee told her he didn't think she was all right and that he was going to help her get outside into the courtyard for fresh air. He gently supported her out of the chair and asked her to slow down her breathing, counting to three on each inhalation and again on each exhalation. When Laura sat down on the bench in the courtyard she started to feel better. She felt very tired and Mr Lee offered to reschedule their meeting and call her a cab so she could go home to rest. In retrospect, Laura understood that she'd suffered a panic attack that had been triggered by her fear of closed-in spaces, also known as claustrophobia.

Starting to support someone with panic attacks

As we can see, the symptoms and causes of panic attacks vary greatly between people. The most common causes are anxiety and stress that don't seem to go away, low mood (depression), fear of specific situations (such as public speaking), the side effects of certain medications and occasionally an effect of poor sleeping habits, recreational drug use or alcohol misuse. Some of these may be relevant to your friend's or relative's own experience of panic attacks, although other causes may also have contributed.

For some people it's not always immediately clear what the sources of causes of their panic attacks are. They may either be unaware of them or ashamed or embarrassed to talk about them. For this reason, when talking to your friend or relative it's important to remember that he or she may not feel able to give you details of some aspects of their personal life; may not even know the causes of their attacks. Consequently, while it may be a useful point of enquiry, don't dwell on finding 'the cause' of the attacks. By all means enquire whether he or she is aware of anything that may be causing them, but don't jump to conclusions – yours or your friend's or relative's. Although you may want to explain why your friend or relative is panicking, you may not spot everything that's having an influence, and it's generally best not to try to offer your own explanations or diagnosis.

It may be useful for both of you to understand what happens when your friend or relative becomes anxious or panicky. You might ask the questions listed here.

- Are there any specific situations that you fear?
- What happens to you when you think about these situations?
- Is there anything in particular that you think makes these situations especially difficult?
- What have you tried to do to solve or avoid this difficulty?
- What's helped – has anything made you more or less anxious?

Don't be afraid to ask your friend or relative how he or she would like you to give support.

We sometimes assume that we know what a partner, close friend or family member needs. This can lead to misunderstandings, even if our actions are carried out with the best intentions. One person, for example, may prefer to be accompanied during an anxiety-provoking situation or receive close support while having a panic attack; someone else may prefer to face a challenge on their own or to have some physical distance from others. What's useful for one individual may not be so for another. You're more likely to be genuinely helpful if you and the person who suffers with panic attacks work together to establish how much or how little he or she would want you to be involved, and how best to react when your friend or relative does have a panic attack.

There's a great deal of useful information in books and online about anxiety and panic attacks – naturally we hope this book will help consolidate much of that. Take the time to learn as much as you can about the condition, how it manifests and how best to treat or manage it. This can be a helpful way of letting someone know you're interested and that you want to help. Similarly, acknowledging that you know your partner, friend, child or relative experiences panic attacks can be validating and supportive. As we've said already, lightly dismissing the person or telling him or her to 'snap out of it' will have the opposite effect/make matters worse, whereas positive, encouraging and supportive behaviours can help remove or relieve feelings of shame or embarrassment – which can in itself be therapeutic. There's no reason panic attacks should simply be accepted as a matter of course and as part of someone's 'personality'.

Gerry was promoted to senior accounts executive at a leading advertising agency. While he welcomed this, he was aware it would require him to pitch to potential clients and sell the company. This would entail public speaking, something he'd been uncomfortable with since his schooldays. As a child he remembered being in the school play and then suddenly forgetting his lines. He was overcome with embarrassment and felt ashamed in front of an audience of parents and other pupils. He became so anxious that as soon as he left the stage, he had palpitations, started to feel nauseous and hyperventilated. Later he was sick. Ever since, Gerry did everything he could to avoid situations where he might have to speak in public. He had a range of excuses to get out of it, and even had to take medication to calm himself before job interviews. Other people close to him who knew of his fear put it down to 'a shy personality', although his therapist explained to him that in the one-to-one context of counselling sessions he didn't present as someone excessively shy. Instead, she explained that as a result of the unfortunate incident at school, he'd learnt to avoid certain stressful situations where he might be prone to panic. Through counselling, he was able to gain confidence in speaking in public, and while he still became anxious, it didn't escalate into full-blown panic attacks.

As we've seen, many people who have panic attacks may feel there's little they can do to change how they feel. Unfortunately this, along with feelings of being out of control, shame, fear and embarrassment, may make them reluctant to seek professional help. If this is the case, listen to their concerns if they're willing and motivated to share them, and encourage them to speak to their GP, who'll offer advice or encouragement and possibly referral to a psychologist, counsellor or psychotherapist. You could also offer to speak to a professional on their behalf to find the best way to get help – though putting pressure on them to get help could make them feel more anxious and delay or even prevent it happening. Nonetheless, it's important to stress that there are effective ways to treat panic attacks and that you're willing to help them find professional help.

Remember that encouraging someone who suffers from panic attacks to seek professional help doesn't mean either of you has failed. It may be that the most supportive thing you can do is to help a friend or relative recognize the huge step he or she has made in asking for help, and support the person in telling his or her story to a GP, counsellor or psychologist.

The frustrating thing about panic attacks

When a close friend or relative has experienced panic attacks on and off for a long period of time, he or she may have developed habits over the months or years that reinforce the situation. It's also possible that you have also developed ways of trying to help them, some less helpful and effective than others. A friend, for example, may encourage someone who experiences panic attacks to consume alcohol before giving an important speech, as a way to steady the nerves. Initially, this may seem a good way to help someone cope with stressful situations, but it merely reinforces the idea that alcohol should precede exposure to them, and alcohol could inadvertently later increase anxiety. Similarly, we might advise our friends or relatives to avoid situations that can trigger extreme anxiety and panic attacks – or go further and offer to do the shopping, say, if that's something that's brought on panic attacks before. We're helping them avoid exposure to the situation they'd find challenging and stressful, which will merely maintain and possibly reinforce the problem, and doesn't allow them to put themselves in a situation where they can test out ideas and skills such as those described in this book. It also encourages reliance and dependency on others to bypass difficult situations. Occasionally, this may be necessary in the short term, but it's not an effective way of treating and overcoming the problem in the long term.

A further example is in the workplace, should we offer to do a presentation on behalf of a colleague who experiences anxiety when undertaking public speaking. Although we're trying to help our colleague feel more comfortable and not be exposed to unpleasant situations, this will do little to advance the colleague's career or treat and overcome his or her difficulties with public speaking. The individual self-confidence won't improve and the same problems will recur.

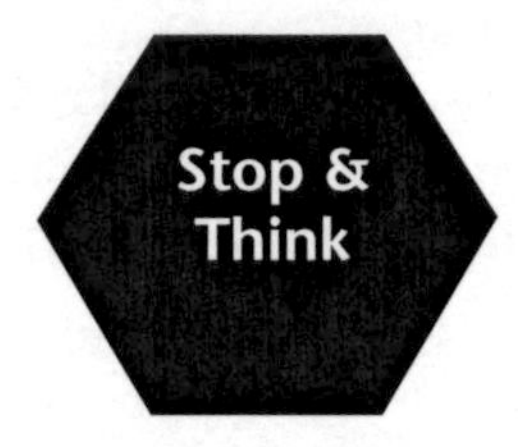

Can you think of any habits you've developed that are helpful to your friend or relative? Are they really helpful or do they prevent that person confronting his or her anxiety and panic attacks? If you discover that you've developed ways of supporting your friend or relative that aren't helpful, gradually stop doing them. This will ensure that you're not enabling that person to use safety behaviours, which are likely to reinforce anxiety in the longer term. It's best to explain first what you're doing and why, so that together you can plan the easiest way to stop reinforcing your friend's or relative's difficulties.

Learning to strike a balance between enabling avoidance and being sensitive to the need for progress is a difficult task for most people. It requires patience and understanding from both the person who has panic attacks and anyone trying to give support. If you find yourself in a situation where a friend or relative is experiencing acute anxiety and suffers a panic attack, stay calm and ask him or her to use some of the relaxation and breathing exercises described in this book.

Seeing someone you care about in acute distress can be very upsetting and leave you feeling helpless and scared yourself. Perhaps the first thing to remember is that acute anxiety generally doesn't last very long. Most people will calm down to a great extent within a maximum of 30 minutes, although the period may seem longer to you. Sometimes bouts of extreme anxiety last moments, and considerably less than half an hour. If you're responsible for someone in acute distress, reminding yourself that it will be over soon may help you stay calm. The most helpful thing you can do is keep the person safe, move him or her to somewhere more private and comfortable if you can, and offer support in finding further sources of help if necessary. Try not to become 'infected' with the same stress and anxiety.

Supporting you as a helper

Another important thing to consider is that the effects of panic attacks can be as challenging to a partner, family member or friend as they are to the person who has them. It's also important to consider support for yourself, because how you cope is likely to influence how he or she copes and vice versa. When it comes to coping with panic attacks, or indeed with most other forms of psychological difficulty, the state of our family relationships as well as how our partners or close friends adapt to the situation may matter more to us than anything else. When close relationships come to feel tense, strained, emotionally distant or volatile, these changes can tip the balance and make us susceptible to increased anxiety, depression and hopelessness, and even worse. An understanding of how relationships can be affected paves the way for more open communication and improved support, both of which have been linked to more favourable health outcomes.

11

Some final thoughts

Having read through this book, you should feel better equipped to understand and cope with panic attacks. At the very least you should have gained insight into their multiple causes or triggers, what physical and cognitive effects they have on us and some specific methods for overcoming them. Self-help may not be all that's required. As we've pointed out, it's sometimes necessary to seek more specialist help and advice from a trained professional, such as a GP, psychologist, counsellor or therapist, whose expertise will certainly be useful and may be needed to make further progress. Remind yourself that you've already made considerable inroads into treating your problem by gaining knowledge and developing insights here. This is an important step in treatment and ultimate recovery. Change, however, takes time, and few people experience instant and complete relief from panic attacks on the basis of having read a book or a single consultation with a therapist. It sometimes takes several weeks or longer for the problem to disappear completely.

We wish you luck on the rest of the journey!

Appendix
How to manage a panic attack while it occurs

Concentrate on managing your panic attack – work through this checklist or use a technique that works for you.

1 Find a quiet place and loosen any tight clothing to make yourself feel more comfortable.
2 Look ahead – focus on an object in front of you.
3 Start to manage your panic by using controlled breathing – gently and slowly breathe in and out.
4 If you're hyperventilating (over-breathing), breathing into a paper bag will help slow your breathing down.
5 Clench your fists very tightly for five seconds and then relax them for five seconds – keep repeating this.
6 If there's someone nearby who's sympathetic and knows about your panic attacks, talk to them.
7 Remind yourself that the panic attack will go in time and is usually over within a couple of minutes.
8 Refocus your attention outside of yourself, for example on what you can see, hear, smell, or on other aspects of your environment.
9 Remember that this is a panic attack – your body will calm down and restabilize soon. You're helping this to happen sooner with these techniques – and you're not going mad, though it can feel like it.

If you've experienced a panic attack, allow yourself time to recuperate, even if it's only for ten minutes or so. Splash cold water on your face; go for a walk to get some fresh air. Also, your blood sugar may be slightly low after a panic attack because of the energy it takes to work through the situation, so try to eat something that's rich in carbohydrates (but avoid too much sugar). Make a note of the techniques you used to manage your panic that were effective – you might want to carry it with you to remind you in future.

When you're feeling more settled, think about whether you should make an appointment with your GP or a therapist to gain an understanding of what might have caused the panic attack and how to prevent or overcome future ones, should they occur.

Other sources of help

If you need more than can be offered by a self-help book, you might like to work with a psychologist or counsellor. We can be contacted via our website: <www.dccclinical.com>

Other sources of psychologists include the following:

British Association for Behavioural and Cognitive Psychotherapies (BABCP)
Imperial House
Hornby Street
Bury
Lancashire BL9 5BN
Tel.: 0161 705 4304
Website: www.babcp.com

British Association for Counselling and Psychotherapy (BACP)
BACP House
15 St John's Business Park
Lutterworth
Leicestershire LE17 4HB
Tel.: 01455 883300
Website: www.bacp.co.uk

British Psychological Society
St Andrew's House
48 Park Road East
Leicester LE1 7DR
Tel.: 0116 254 9568
Website: www.bps.org.uk

Health and Care Professions Council
Park House
184 Kennington Park Road
London SE11 4BU
Tel.: 0845 300 6184
Website: www.hpc-uk.org

These associations all set standards for membership and their websites offer a search facility to find a therapist near you. If you want to know that a psychologist who has been recommended is registered with the Health and Care Professions Council in the UK, its website allows you to check this. Your GP will also be able to put you in touch with reputable local professionals.

Index